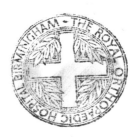

Joint Replacement in the Shoulder and Elbow

Joint Replacement in the Shoulder and Elbow

Edited by

W. Angus Wallace FRCSEd, FRCS(Orth)
Professor of Orthopaedic and Accident Surgery, University of Nottingham;
Consultant Orthopaedic Surgeon, Queen's Medical Centre,
Nottingham, previously Harlow Wood Orthopaedic Hospital, Nr Mansfield, UK
and now the Nottingham Shoulder and Elbow Unit, City Hospital, Nottingham, UK

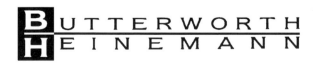

OXFORD   BOSTON   JOHANNESBURG   MELBOURNE   NEW DELHI   SINGAPORE

Butterworth-Heinemann
Linacre House, Jordan Hill, Oxford OX2 8DP
225 Wildwood Avenue, Woburn, MA 01801-2041
A division of Reed Educational and Professional Publishing Ltd

℞ A member of the Reed Elsevier plc group

First published 1998

British Library Cataloguing in Publication Data
Joint replacement in the shoulder and elbow
  1. Artificial joints   2. Arm – Surgery
  I. Wallace, W. A.
  617/5'7

Library of Congress Cataloguing in Publication Data
Joint replacement in the shoulder and elbow/edited by W. Angus Wallace
  p. cm.
  Includes bibliographical references and index.
  ISBN 0 7506 1367 X
  1   Artificial shoulder joints.   2   Total elbow replacement.
  I   Wallace, W. Angus.
  [DNLM: 1   Shoulder Joint–surgery.   2   Joint Prosthesis.   3   Elbow
  Joint–surgery. WE 810 J74]
  RD557.5.J65
  617.5'720592–dc21   97–30915
                                                                                          CIP

ISBN 0 7506 1367 X

Typeset by Bath Typesetting Ltd
Printed and bound in Great Britain at the Bath Press, Avon

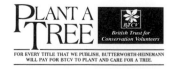

Contents

Contributors

Andrew A. Amis PhD, CEng, FIMechE
Reader in Orthopaedic Biomechanics,
Imperial College, London, UK

Christopher R. Constant LLM, MCh, FRCS
Consultant Orthopaedic Surgeon,
Specialist in Shoulder and Elbow Surgery,
Department of Trauma and Orthopaedic Surgery,
Addenbrooke's Hospital, Cambridge, UK

Dorcas Damrel MCSP
Senior Physiotherapist, previously Harlow Wood
Orthopaedic Hospital, Nr Mansfield, UK and now the Nottingham
Shoulder and Elbow Unit, City Hospital,
Nottingham, UK

Philip Hirst FRCS
Consultant Orthopaedic Surgeon,
Manchester Royal Infirmary,
Manchester, UK

Ian G. Kelly BSc, MD, FRCS(Ed) FRCPS (Glas)
Consultant Orthopaedic Surgeon,
Orthopaedic Directorate,
Royal Infirmary, Glasgow, UK

Peter G. Lunn FRCS
Consultant Orthopaedic and Hand Surgeon,
Derbyshire Royal Infirmary, Derby, UK

Thomas R. Redfern MChOrth, FRCS(Ed)
Consultant Orthopaedic Surgeon,
Leighton Hospital, Crewe, UK

John K. Stanley
Professor of Upper Limb Surgery and
Consultant Orthopaedic Surgeon,
Wrightington Hospital, Nr Wigan, UK

W. Angus Wallace FRCS(Ed) & Eng, FRCS(Orth)
Professor of Orthopaedic and Accident Surgery,
University of Nottingham;
Consultant Orthopaedic Surgeon, Queen's Medical Centre,
previously Harlow Wood Orthopaedic Hospital, Nr Mansfield, UK
and now the Nottingham Shoulder and Elbow Unit, City Hospital, Nottingham, UK

Introduction

W. Angus Wallace

Starting off in shoulder surgery in the 1970s in Britain

Shoulder surgery was a Cinderella specialty in the UK in the 1970s. The only common shoulder operations were for recurrent anterior dislocation of the shoulder; the standard operation used was the Putti–Platt operation – probably invented by Putti at the Rizzoli Institute, Bologna, Italy but brought to the UK by Platt and popularized by Osmond-Clarke (1948) with his article on 'Habitual dislocation of the shoulder. The Putti–Platt operation'.

Very few orthopaedic surgeons in the UK understood many of the shoulder pathologies and the author had his interest in the shoulder stimulated by attending a training course on 'Examination of the musculoskeletal system' run by James Cyriax of St Thomas's Hospital, London in 1977. Following this a research project on shoulder movement was carried out in Nottingham as a result of a Medical Research Council Training Research Fellowship and this has led to a lifetime interest in the shoulder and more recently in the elbow.

Milestones in the development of shoulder replacement surgery

The history and development of shoulder replacement are described in Chapter 1 but a brief résumé of shoulder arthroplasty develop-ment is appropriate here. Shoulder replacement was pioneered in the 1950s with several prosthetic replacements designed for the upper part of the humerus. These included acrylic prostheses (Edelmann, 1951; Van der Ghinst and Houssa, 1951; Richard, Judet and René, 1952) and cobalt chrome prostheses (Krueger, 1951; Neer, Brown and McLaughlin, 1953). Of these prostheses, the Neer hemiarthroplasty, developed by Dr Charles Neer II in New York (Figure 1), became the most popular, particu-larly for four-part fractures but also for diseases in which articular cartilage is destroyed but in which there is no distortion of the glenoid subchondral bone (Neer, 1974). In the early 1970s several investigators developed con-strained designs of total replacement prostheses for the shoulder. These included the Stanmore total shoulder replacement (TSR) developed by Lettin and Scales in London, the Kölbel TSR in Germany, the Leeds TSR developed by Reeves, the Liverpool TSR developed by Cavendish and Elloy, the Bickel TSR developed at the Mayo Clinic in the USA, and finally the Kessel TSR developed in London. The Bickel was first used in 1972 and went through a very popular honeymoon period. Unfortunately it became clear by the late 1970s that constrained designs resulted in unacceptable loosening rates. In 1977 the Institution of Mechanical Engineers in London held a unique Conference on Joint Replacement in the Upper Limb, in which the problems relating to the newer joint replace-ments were highlighted, and the papers from that meeting were published in the Conference

Proceedings (Institution of Mechanical Engineers, 1977). Over the subsequent 10 years constrained shoulder replacements were gradually abandoned. In 1972 Averill and Neer also developed three fixed fulcrum prostheses but active movement with their devices was disappointing and they were abandoned (Neer, Watson and Stanton, 1982). In 1973 Neer modified his hemiarthroplasty and introduced a glenoid component which was anchored with polymethylmethacrylate bone cement. This has proved to be the most popular prosthesis in use worldwide and by 1982 Neer and his colleagues were able to report the results of 273 consecutive shoulders treated with their design of prosthesis (Neer, Watson and Stanton, 1982). By 1990 there had been sufficient experience of total shoulder replacement to assess the complication rates and the need for revision surgery. Careful analytical work by Cofield and Edgerton (1990) highlighted the problems of glenoid loosening, dislocation and rotator cuff tears. Different designs of prosthesis have been introduced to address some of these problems, with the Cofield TSR introduced at the Mayo Clinic in 1986, the biomodular introduced by Dines and Warren at the Hospital for Special Surgery, New York in 1987 and the Nottingham introduced by Wallace in 1994. All these designs have attempted to improve on what continues to be the gold standard – the Neer II TSR, against which all these new designs should be evaluated.

Milestones in the development of elbow replacement surgery

Total elbow replacement (TER) has followed a similar pattern of development to TSR. This is covered in more detail in Chapter 8. Initially the constrained TERs were introduced in the 1960s by Dee from New York, and subsequently the Stanmore and the St Georg were developed. Next the semiconstrained metal-to-plastic hinges were popularized in the USA, particularly in the 1970s, with the introduction of the Coonrad and Pritchard–Walker prostheses. However, a significant milestone was the publication by Souter of his paper on 'Arthroplasty of the elbow with particular reference to metallic hinge arthroplasty in rheumatoid patients' in 1973 (Souter, 1973) which high-

lighted the prob-lems of the hinged prostheses and made a plea for designs with less in-built constraint. The need for such less constrained prostheses became clear at the Conference on Joint Replacement in the Upper Limb (Institution of Mechanical Engineers, 1977), at which the problems of hinged replacements were openly discussed. Souter subsequently developed the Souter–Strathclyde TER with collaboration from Paul and Nicoll at Strathclyde University. A different design of unconstrained elbow replacement (the Kudo TER) was developed by Kudo at Sagamihara National Hospital in Japan, and both the Souter–Strathclyde and the Kudo have become the preferred TERs in the UK in 1997, as highlighted in Chapter 10.

Triennial International Conference on Surgery of the Shoulder (ICSS)

We owe a debt of gratitude to Lipmann Kessel who, with Ian Bayley at the Royal National Orthopaedic Hospital in London, realized that the time had come to bring shoulder surgeons from all over the world together for an International Conference on Surgery of the Shoulder. The first meeting was held in London in 1980. Great efforts, particularly by Ian Bayley, resulted in the publication shortly afterwards of the majority of the papers presented at the meeting in *Shoulder Surgery* (Bayley and Kessel, 1982). This set the pattern for the next 9 years. The 2nd ICSS was held in Toronto in 1983 and hosted by James Bateman and Peter Welsh. The papers from that meeting were published in *Surgery of the Shoulder* (Bateman and Welsh, 1984). The 3rd ICSS was held in Fukuoka, Japan in 1986 and was hosted by Nahoto Takagishi. The papers from that meeting were published in *The Shoulder* (Takagishi, 1987). The 4th ICSS had been planned for San Fransisco, with the Chairman to have been Robert Samilson but regrettably he died shortly after the plans for the meeting were laid. Therefore Charles Neer and Charlie Rockwood organized the 4th ICSS in New York in 1989. By this stage the Conference had become a large international meeting and it became impractical to continue publishing the papers from the meeting as a separate publication. This decision was further influenced by the emergence of the *Journal of Shoulder and Elbow Surgery* – an international publication which is

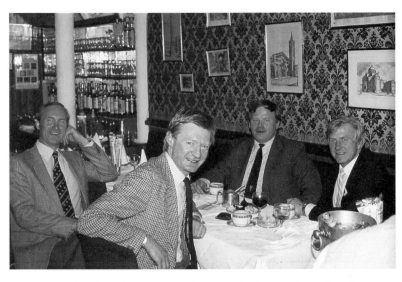

Figure 1 The founding members of the British Elbow and Shoulder Society.

now firmly established. In 1992 the 5th ICSS was held in Paris. Originally it had been planned that Didier Patte, who had an outstanding reputation as a shoulder surgeon, would have been Chairman but regrettably he died the year before the meeting; and Daniel Goutallier was selected as the Chairman of the Conference, with a team of three (André Apoil, Michel Mansat and Gilles Walch) working together as the Organizing Committee. In 1995 the 6th ICSS was held in Helsinki, Finland (host Martii Vastamaki) and in Stockholm, Sweden (host Richard Wallenstein).

British Elbow and Shoulder Society (BESS)

The British Elbow and Shoulder Society was founded as a result of an increasing interest in shoulder and elbow surgery in the UK in the early 1980s, and particularly after a very successful Third ICSS meeting in Japan. The stimulus came from Michael Watson, who wrote the following letter on 3 November 1986:

> I think the time has come to take the bull by the horns and seriously consider the nuts and bolts of setting up a British Shoulder Surgery Association. I am sure that we are going to start to get enquiries for our corporate stance on technical and administrative features of shoulder surgery and it would be difficult to

establish a common attitude without an association.

> I suggest an organisation under the umbrella of the BOA with the approval of you and the others who were in Japan (3rd ICSS). I propose that we get the ball rolling.

As a result of that letter the founding members of BESS (Michael Watson, Ian Bayley, Steve Copeland and the author) met on 28 March 1987 at 92 Harley Street in London (Figure 1) and set up the Society. The meetings of BESS have been held annually and are listed in Table 1. It was an honour for the author to be appointed the Treasurer of the Society for its first 5 years.

Société Européene pour la Chirurgie de l'Epaule et du Coude (SECEC) (European Society for Surgery of the Shoulder and the Elbow (ESSSE))

The Society was founded by Didier Patte from Melun in France who was a world authority on shoulder surgery, particularly repair of rotator cuff tears, and Norbert Gschwend who had been a leader in rheumatoid arthritis and joint replacement surgery. The meetings of the Society started as annual events but now, every 3 years, the meeting is not held in order to accommodate the meetings of the International

Table 1 Meetings of the British Elbow and Shoulder Society

Meeting	Venue and date	Chairman
Inaugural	Glasgow, March 1988	Ian Kelly, Western Infirmary, Glasgow
1st	Edinburgh, March 1989	Willie Souter, Princess Margaret Rose Hospital, Edinburgh
2nd	London, March 1990	Ian Bayley, Stanmore (Royal National Orthopaedic Hospital), London
3rd	Liverpool, March 1991	Howard Beddow, Royal Liverpool Hospital, Liverpool
4th	Exeter, April 1992	Tim Bunker, Princess Elizabeth Orthopaedic Hospital, Exeter
5th	Manchester, March 1993	Clive Warren-Smith, Wythenshawe Hospital, Manchester
6th	London, February 1994	Michael Watson, Guy's Hospital, London
7th	Reading, September 1995	Steve Copeland, Reading University
8th	Dublin, May 1997	James Colville, Dublin

Table 2 Meetings of the Société Européene pour la Chirurgie de l'Epaule et du Coude

Meeting	Venue and date	Chairman/Chairmen
1st Inaugural	Paris, France November 1987	Didier Patte, Melun, France Norbert Gschwend, Zurich, Switzerland
2nd	Berne, Switzerland September/October 1988	Didier Patte, Melun, France Christian Gerber, Berne, Switzerland
3rd	New York, USA October 1989	Business meeting only at 4th ICSS (Charles Neer and Charles Rockwood)
4th	Milan, Italy October 1990	Mario Randelli, Milan, Italy
5th	Wurzburg, Germany June 1991	Joacquim Eulert, Wurzburg, Germany
6th	Paris, France July 1992	Business meeting only at 5th ICSS (Daniel Goutallier)
7th	Aarhus, Denmark June 1993	Otto Sneppen, Aarhus, Denmark
8th	Barcelona, Spain June 1994	Joachim Poal-Manresa, Barcelona, Spain
9th	Nottingham, England September 1996	Angus Wallace, Nottingham, England
10th	Salzburg, Austria September 1997	Herbert Resch, Salzburg, Austria

Conference of Surgery of the Shoulder (ICSS). The meetings with their venues and dates are shown in Table 2.

Journal of Shoulder and Elbow Surgery (JSES)

The success of the International Conferences on Surgery of the Shoulder had highlighted the degree of international interest that there was in shoulder surgery. At the 4th ICSS in New York a new journal was planned: the *Journal of Shoulder and Elbow Surgery*. Dr Charles Neer in New York devoted the last few years of his working life before retirement in setting up the journal, and although he had decided from an early stage that he did not wish to take on the Editorship, he remains Chairman of the Founding Board of Trustees and considers the journal as one of his progeny.

Dr Robert Cofield from the Mayo Clinic was elected Editor-in-Chief succeeded by Bob Neviaser in 1997. There is a team of Editors working with them from all over the world: Rich Hawkins and Andrew Weiland from North America; Michel Mansat from France, as European Editor, with Ian Kelly from Scotland as Co-Editor for Europe; Kosaku Mizuno from Japan; Arnaldo Ferreira from Brazil; David Sonnabend from Australia; and Donald Mackenzie from South Africa.

The journal began publication in 1992 and during that year over 100 manuscripts were submitted. By 1997 the effect of the journal has been to stimulate clinical and scientific research into shoulder and elbow surgery and as a consequence an increased flow of submitted papers ensured that only papers of good quality were being published.

The future

Total shoulder replacement is broadly carried out for three indications: rheumatoid arthritis, osteoarthritis (primary or secondary) and malunion after fractures. There is some evidence that new drugs are becoming available that have a significant effect on rheumatoid arthritis, damping down the disease and reducing the amount of resulting bone damage. It is unlikely, however, that these drugs are going to reduce the need for joint replacement in patients with rheumatoid arthritis. However, it does seem that the incidence of rheumatoid arthritis in the UK is beginning to fall. The reasons for this are not clear but epidemiological studies are currently being carried out to investigate whether this is an accurate observation.

In relation to osteoarthritis we are going to see a significant increase in symptomatic osteoarthritis of the shoulder over the next 10 years. This is because of the enlarging elderly population and the fact that the elderly nowadays are expecting a much more active retirement than they have been in the past. Requests for shoulder replacement from family doctors are very likely to increase significantly.

In relation to fracture treatment, early intervention with reduction and fixation (either open or closed) is being carried out but a significant number of patients are being missed and late malunion with symptoms remains a significant problem. Although the author believes that there will be an improvement in primary management of humeral neck fractures, it is anticipated that the numbers that are presenting with symptomatic malunions are likely to increase.

In relation to elbow replacement, the success over the last 10 years of both the Souter–Strathclyde and the Kudo minimally constrained elbow replacements means that they are likely to be used more generally in the future. Already papers are appearing on the use of elbow replacement after severe fracture malunion but there remains a real concern about using elbow replacement for osteoarthritis when the osteoarthritis has often been brought on by heavy manual work. Loosening of the com-ponents of the elbow replacement remains the worrying long-term risk, however the author believes that, certainly in the UK, the number of elbow replacements being carried out annually is likely to double over the next 5 years.

The surgeon has a responsibility to train himself or herself to provide the best possible technical operation and to minimize the complications from joint replacement with a good fixation technique and a low incidence of primary infection. If these are maintained then joint replacement of the shoulder and elbow will begin to develop the same reputation for success as joint replacement in the lower limb. It is hoped that this volume will help the surgeon with the selection of patients and the technical aspects of their surgical treatment, as well as giving guidance on postoperative physiotherapy treatment.

References

Bateman JE and Welsh RP (eds) 1984) *Surgery of the Shoulder*. Philadelphia: Becker

Bayley I and Kessel L (eds) (1982) *Shoulder Surgery*. Berlin: Springer.

Edelman G (1951) Traitment immédiat des fractures complexes de l'extrémité supérieure de l'humérus par prothèse acrylique. *Presse Médicale* **59** 1777–1778.

Institution of Mechanical Engineers (1977) *Proceedings of the Conference on Joint Replacement of the Upper Limb*. London: IMechE.

Krueger FJ (1951) Vitallium replica arthroplasty of the shoulder: a case report of aseptic necrosis of the proximal end of the humerus. *Surgery* **301** 1005–1011.

Neer CS II (1974) Replacement arthroplasty for glenohumeral osteoarthritis. *Journal of Bone and Joint Surgery* **56A** 1–13.

Neer CS, Brown TH and McLaughlin HL (1953) Fractures of the neck of the humerus with dislocation of the head fragment. *American Journal of Surgery* **85** 252–258.

Neer CS II, Watson KC and Stanton FJ (1982) Recent experience in total shoulder replacement. *Journal of Bone and Joint Surgery* **63A** 319–337.

Osmond-Clarke H (1948) Habitual dislocation of the shoulder. The Putti–Platt operation. *Journal of Bone and Joint Surgery* **30B** 19–25.

Richard A, Judet R and René L (1952) Reconstruction prothétique acrylique de l'extrémité supérieure de l'humérus spécialement au cours des fractures-luxations. *Journal de Chirurgie* **68** 537–547.

Souter WA (1973) Arthroplasty of the elbow – with particular reference to metallic hinge arthroplasty in rheumatoid patients. *Orthopaedic Clinics of North America* **4** 395–413.

Takagishi N (ed.) (1987) *The Shoulder*. Proceedings of the 3rd International Conference on Surgery of the Shoulder. Fukuoka, Japan: Professional Postgraduate Services.

Van der Ghinst M and Houssa P (1951) Prothèses acryliques et fractures de l'extrémité supérieure des membres. *Acta Chirurgica Belgica* **42** 31–40.

1

History of shoulder replacement surgery

Thomas R. Redfern and W. Angus Wallace

Shoulder prostheses in the late nineteenth century

During the late nineteenth century, animal bone and ivory were used for the fabrication of prostheses for use in humans. A pioneer of this work was the Frenchman Gluck, who was recorded by Péan in 1894 as the first person to design and construct a prosthetic shoulder. There is no record of its successful use.

The first fully documented glenohumeral arthroplasty was performed by the outstanding French Surgeon, Jules Emile Péan (1894). In 1893 a 37-year-old Parisian baker named Jules Perdoux consulted Péan for treatment of a suppurating tuberculous left shoulder. Péan recommended forequarter amputation, which Perdoux declined, and so he performed a thorough debridement of soft tissue and bone instead. Péan's technician, Mathieu, designed a prosthesis along the lines of the Gluck prosthesis, but Péan feared this would be too weak and would limit shoulder movement. He approached a dentist, Dr J. Porter Michaels, who had previously fabricated a maxillary prosthesis of platinum for him. Michaels quickly designed and made a prosthesis with a platinum shaft with transverse holes placed distally for screw fixation to the humeral shaft, and two longitudinal ridges drilled more proximally with small holes to allow for the reattachment of muscles. At its upper end the prosthesis comprised a rubber ball boiled in paraffin for 24 hours to render it stable to tissue fluids. Two thick platinum wires were laid at

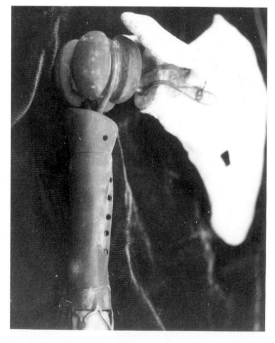

Figure 1.1 The Péan shoulder. (Reproduced with kind permission of Mr Alan Hawk, Historical Collections, National Museum of Health and Medicine, Armed Forces Institute of Pathology, Washington, DC.)

right angles to each other in deep circumferential grooves, one being screwed to the side of the glenoid and the other attached to the platinum shaft (Figure 1.1).

This prosthesis was inserted by Péan using an anterior approach to the shoulder. Twelve days later the patient was allowed up and he was discharged home on the 20th postoperative day.

Discharge from recurrent fistulae along the line of the surgical scar persisted but Perdoux was pain-free and recovered from the systemic effects of tuberculosis. Two years later, when the fistulae had become increasingly troublesome and when radiographs showed a shell of new bone around the joint, the prosthesis was removed. Perdoux gradually recovered and returned to work, and the prosthesis is now on display in the Smithsonian Institute in Washington, DC (Lugli, 1978).

Early twentieth century – reconstruction without prostheses

There are no further reports of prosthetic glenohumeral arthroplasties until the 1950s. The incidence of tuberculosis gradually declined during the early part of the twentieth century but the Great War produced new patients with gross glenohumeral joint destruction, most of whom were victims of gunshot and shrapnel wounds. These were often treated by excision arthroplasty of the glenohumeral joint.

A method of humeral head reconstruction using a free fibula graft in patients with an intact rotator cuff was described by Rovsing in 1910, Skillern in 1920 and Albee in 1921. In 1933, Lawrence Jones described a reconstruction of the glenohumeral joint in which the rotator cuff muscles were inserted into the rounded end of the proximal humerus after resection of the humeral head. Although his results were spectacular, others were unable to repeat them and the operation soon lost popularity.

Hemiarthroplasties

In the early 1950s there was a sudden resurgence of interest in prostheses for the glenohumeral joint, particularly humeral head replacements. Krueger (1951) reported the use of a cobalt chrome prosthesis for an avascular humeral head in a seaman. Richard, Judet and Rene used an acrylic prosthesis similar to the famous Judet hip for hip fracture patients, reporting their work in 1952. Other workers also used an acrylic prosthesis for the humeral head in fracture cases (Edelmann, 1951; van der Ghinst and Houssa, 1951).

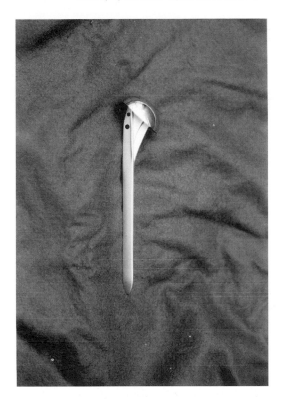

Figure 1.2 The Neer Mark I prosthesis. (Courtesy of Homedica International Ltd.)

In New York, Dr Charles Neer II had become disillusioned with the conventional methods of managing complicated fractures and fracture dislocations of the humeral head. His Mark I humeral head replacement was first reported in 1953 (Neer, Brown and McLaughlin, 1953) and in 1955 the clinical results of his first 18 patients were published (Neer, 1955). The vitallium Neer Mark I prosthesis was a simple hollow hemisphere mounted on a stem with three flanges, each drilled with multiple holes to facilitate the anchorage of the rotator cuff and its bony attachments. Good pain relief and a satisfactory return of shoulder function were reported. Neer continued his pioneering work and by 1974 (Neer, 1974) had added 48 patients to his series. He had used his prosthesis for osteoarthritis and avascular necrosis (Figure 1.2).

Hemiarthroplasties were also developed by several workers for the treatment of proximal humeral tumours. Those of Ducci (1963), Lynn, Alexakis and Bechtol (1965) and Casuccio (1966) did not permit reconstruction of the rotator cuff and the proximal humeral musculature. Haraldsson addressed this problem and described his 'muscle sling prosthesis' in 1969. Despite efforts to reconstruct the soft tissues, elevation beyond horizontal was not achieved. There are no further reports of the use of this prosthesis and a long-stemmed Neer prosthesis will achieve a similar result after proximal humeral resection.

Macnab (1977) reported the experimental development and use of an uncemented bipolar shoulder prosthesis. Good clinical results were obtained, but in rotator cuff-deficient patients upward subluxation was a problem, causing loss of both rotation and abduction. Acromionectomy was reported sometimes to resolve this problem. Some 2 years earlier (in 1975), Monk in Liverpool used a modification of his 'hard-topped' bipolar hip prosthesis in one patient. The clinical result was poor and was not reported in the literature.

Swanson (1984) reported the use of a bipolar hemiarthroplasty for the shoulder. This prosthesis comprised a humeral stem supporting a 26 mm sphere. This was enclosed by an outer head of 38, 43 or 48 mm. The prosthesis was designed to articulate with the glenoid and to transmit load, through the rotator cuff, to the acromion and the coracoacromial ligament. It was self-centring and brought the centre of rotation away from the coracoacromial arch. It was stable, easy to insert, could be used as a revision after glenoid component failure in other prostheses and was designed to decrease stress concentrations and hence decrease pressure on the rotator cuff. Despite these perceived advantages, the design does not appear to have been widely accepted and used by others.

Constrained and semiconstrained prostheses

On both sides of the Atlantic interest in hinged and other constrained shoulder prostheses continued. In the UK, Lettin and Scales (Lettin, 1982), disappointed with the results of the Neer prosthesis in patients with rheumatoid arthritis, described the Stanmore prosthesis which they had designed in conjunction with Goddard and had first used in 1969. The conventional semiconstrained ball and socket design had a deep glenoid socket, and fixation to the surrounding glenoid was enhanced by three metal spikes. They reported the results of

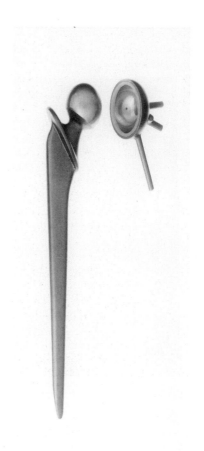

Figure 1.3 The Stanmore prosthesis.

their first two patients to the Royal Society of Medicine in 1971 (Lettin and Scales, 1972) (Figure 1.3).

In the same year, Macnab had designed a semiconstrained prosthesis whose glenoid was porous coated to allow bone ingrowth (Welsh and Macnab, 1985b). A snap-fit polyethylene insert lined the glenoid component, which was extended superiorly to provide an effective fulcrum for abductor function. Gains in movement were considered disappointing and use of the prosthesis was discontinued.

Subsequent papers by Coughlin, Morris and West (1979) in San Francisco and by Lettin, Copeland and Scales (1982) in the UK indicated that loosening of the glenoid component was a major problem with the Stanmore prosthesis. This, and the poor results with the Neer prosthesis in rotator cuff-deficient patients, caused renewed interest in the design of constrained total shoulder arthroplasties.

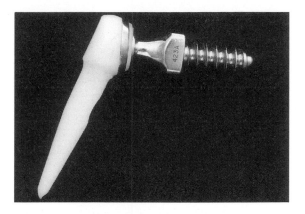

Figure 1.5 The Kessel prosthesis.

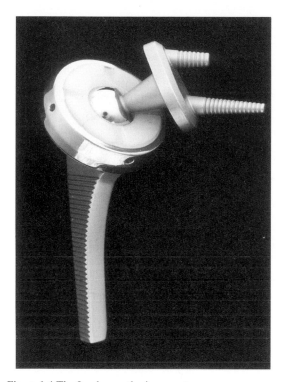

Figure 1.4 The Leeds prosthesis.

Reeves and Jobbins in Leeds reported on their extensive laboratory work in 1972 (Reeves, Jobbins and Flowers, 1972; Reeves et al, 1972a) and in 1973 (Jobbins, Flowers and Reeves, 1973). They had considered three potential designs and 12 methods of glenoid component fixation, including ten designs of pegs for the components. They felt that reversing the anatomy to give a glenoid ball and a socket enclosed in the excavated humeral head restored the anatomical centre of rotation and prevented impingement of the humeral component below the acromion. The resulting wholly constrained Leeds prosthesis (Figure 1.4) was used in a small group of patients with satisfactory early results (Reeves et al, 1972b) although no further reports of its use have been reported in the literature.

In Europe, Kölbel of Berlin adopted the reversed ball and socket design, reporting on his prosthesis in 1975 (Kölbel and Friedebold, 1975). He used a single glenoid peg supplemented by a metal outrigger or flange which was anchored to the scapula at the base of the coracoid by a large screw. This prosthesis and the design principles behind it were discussed further at the 1st International Conference on Surgery of the Shoulder in London in 1980 (Kölbel, Rohlmann and Bergmann, 1982), and modifications to the outrigger were described at the 2nd International Conference in Toronto in 1983 (Kölbel, 1984).

An alternative approach was reported in 1975 by Zippel, who secured a glenoid dish with a central screw supplemented by two metal studs. The design was not adopted elsewhere, perhaps because the reversed ball and socket design had achieved such wide acceptance.

In London, Kessel used the reversed ball and socket configuration, with the glenoid ball being implanted by means of a strong self-tapping lag screw (Kessel and Bayley, 1979) (Figure 1.5). The device had been used in 24 shoulders and the results were satisfactory in most of the first 18 assessed. A subsequent report (Bayley and Kessel, 1982) has suggested that loosening and dislocation have been problems with this prosthesis – problems encountered with all constrained prostheses and not unique to the Kessel design.

In 1977 Beddow and Elloy reported that they had adopted the same reversed ball and socket principle for the semiconstrained Liverpool shoulder (Figure 1.6). The glenoid component comprised a small ball supported by a long curved stem introduced into the axillary border of the scapula. Difficulty in reaming the axillary border of the scapula resulted in a modification with a smaller axillary stem. The prosthesis had been used successfully in nine shoulders and was subsequently used until the mid-1980s, when it was superseded by an unconstrained prosthesis.

Beddow and Elloy (1982) also reported that they had designed the Beddow Mark I pros-

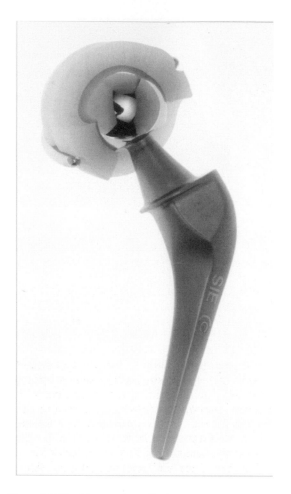

Figure 1.6 The Liverpool prosthesis.

thesis, with a conventional humeral ball and glenoid socket, and again using the axillary border of the scapula for fixation of the glenoid component. This prosthesis was of metal on metal, a combination used by Wheble, Skorecki and Thompson (1977) in Manchester. Their totally constrained prosthesis was tested exhaustively in the laboratory, but was ultimately used in only one patient with a tumour. This prosthesis was unusual in that it was designed for insertion through a posterior approach to the shoulder.

Enormous forces are transmitted through constrained shoulder prostheses (Fenlin, 1975). In general, the tendency for a prosthesis to loosen increases with the degree of constraint, but in two highly constrained prostheses, fracture of the components occurred before glenoid loosening. The first of these, the Bickel prosthesis, was reported by Cofield and

Stauffer (1977) from the Mayo Clinic. It comprised a cobalt chrome-stemmed humeral ball which articulated with two high-density polyethylene hemispheres encased in a cobalt chrome shell which was cemented into the excavated glenoid. Fracture of the prosthetic humeral neck occurred in two of 12 patients, and in a further two shoulders the glenoid fractured, leading to component instability and pain.

The second highly constrained prosthesis was that of Dr Melvin Post in the USA. In 1979 he published results of his first series of 24 prostheses made of stainless steel (Post et al, 1979). Six had suffered fracture of the prosthetic humeral neck, and a further two bent. In a subsequent series manufactured from cobalt chrome, two of 21 components failed. Significantly, no glenoid loosening was encountered in 43 prostheses. Post attributed this to two factors: (1) the prosthesis was designed to dislocate when torque became excessive or the functional range of movement was exceeded; and (2) fixation of the glenoid component was achieved with screws, and therefore without disruption of the subchondral bone plate which Post believed to be essential for satisfactory long-term fixation of constrained prostheses (Post, Haskill and Jablon, 1980). However, in a subsequent paper in 1983 (Post and Jablon, 1983) he reported that complications had occurred with his Series II prosthesis, including eight dislocations, three loose glenoids and two with broken screws in a series of 78 patients.

Two more constrained prostheses were reported in 1978. Each was an attempt to allow the centre of rotation of the prosthesis to change during movement while maintaining full constraint. Buechel, Pappas and DePalma (1978) described their 'floating socket' prosthesis in which a small metal glenoid ball was placed inside a larger polyethylene ball which was enclosed within a metal cup located within the humeral head; satisfactory early results were reported in six patients. Gristina and Webb (1982) described their equally ingenious trispherical prosthesis. This had two metallic spheres (one mounted on the glenoid and the other on the humeral head), linked by a central polyethylene ball containing two sockets. The design has not been successful and neither prosthesis has merited further use.

The plethora of constrained prostheses proves the deficiencies of this type of design.

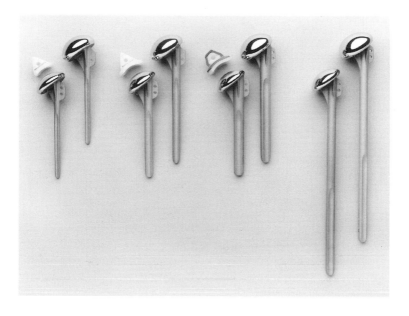

Figure 1.7 The Neer Mark II prosthesis. (Courtesy of 3M Health Care Ltd.)

Dislocations, implant failure and loosening of components have been problems with all constrained and semiconstrained designs, and most have now been rejected. Only the Kessel remains in use although its popularity is declining. A constrained prosthesis for the rotator cuff-deficient patient is still required, but a stable design with a durable glenoid fixation remains an elusive goal.

Unconstrained prostheses

The first unconstrained total shoulder arthroplasty recorded in the literature was that of Kenmore, Maccartee and Brantley (1974). Results with the widely used Neer hemiarthroplasty had not been entirely successful in their hands and in 1972 they sought a glenoid component to create a total shoulder joint arthroplasty. No such component was available in the USA so they developed a 3 mm thick elliptical polypropylene disc with central stem and used this in three patients.

Neer modified his Mark I humeral head in 1973 so that its edges were rounded off and did not impinge at the extremes of movement (Neer, 1974). A high-density polyethylene glenoid component was added and the resulting Neer Mark II prosthesis remains unchanged to date. It is the most commonly used shoulder

prosthesis throughout the world. It is available now in three head sizes, three stem diameters, three stem lengths and with a choice of five glenoid components (Neer, Watson and Stanton, 1982) (Figure 1.7). A metal-backed glenoid was added to the range in the early 1980s following occasional fracture between the articular surface and the keel of high-density polyethylene glenoids in young active patients (Neer, 1984).

In 1974 Stellbrink and Englebrecht designed the St Georg prosthesis (Englebrecht and Stellbrink, 1975). This comprised a 39 mm stemmed humeral sphere articulating with a 32 mm diameter circular glenoid dish with an extended superior lip secured by a central circular peg (Siegel and Englebrecht, 1977; Siegel et al, 1977). Despite this, dislocation and superior subluxation were seen in rotator cuff-deficient patients (Englebrecht, 1984).

Extension of the superior lip of the glenoid component was used by Macnab and English (1976) of Toronto but elevation beyond 110° was not achieved and this prosthesis has not been widely used. Neer also designed glenoid components with extended superior lips. The '200%' and '600%' glenoids were used only rarely for severe rheumatoid arthritis and cuff tear arthropathy. It has become clear that the use of glenoid components with an extended superior lip results in increased constraint of the humeral head and they suffer the same fate as constrained prostheses – glenoid component loosening progressing to failure. They are no longer used.

In 1977 Mathys and Mathys reported on the isoelastic shoulder prosthesis but, as problems on the humeral side of the shoulder are seldom seen, the advantages of this prosthesis over a standard metal-stemmed component have yet to be demonstrated in clinical practice.

Acceptance of the Neer prosthesis increased through the late 1970s but in Los Angeles, Clarke et al (1981) designed a further non-constrained prosthesis. It differed little from the Neer Mark I humeral head, other than in having a tapering stem and an antirotation flange. There were two glenoid options: one elliptical but similar to the Neer glenoid, and the other with a superior extension. Subsequently the keel of the glenoid component was moved inferiorly to avoid superomedial tilting of the component due to the loss of bone stock superiorly in severely damaged glenoids (Amstutz, Sew Hoy and Clarke, 1981).

In the UK, Beddow in Liverpool designed his Mark III prosthesis in 1979. Similar to the St Georg, it is still used with satisfactory results by the designer. The initial central peg of the glenoid component was altered in 1983. It now has two divergent pegs for anchorage into the axillary border of the scapula and into the base of the glenoid (Figure 1.8).

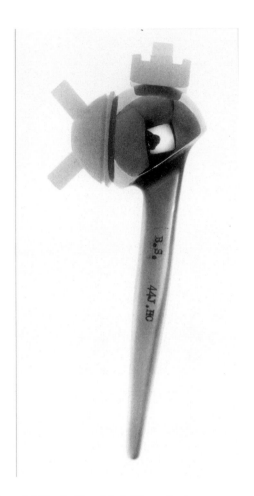

Figure 1.8 The Beddow Mark III prosthesis.

Subacromial spacers

During the late 1970s it became clear that restoration of a satisfactory range of movement in unconstrained shoulders depended on sound repair of the rotator cuff rather than on glenoid component design. In an attempt to improve the results in patients with irreparable rotator cuff tears, three designs of subacromial spacer were introduced. All were intended to hold the humeral head down during the initial stages of abduction, until the remainder of the rotator cuff musculature could stabilize the head while the deltoid continued to produce elevation.

The first was described in 1977 by Welsh and Macnab (1985a). A similar design was developed in Liverpool about the same time and was first reported in 1982 (Beddow and Elloy, 1982) (Figure 1.8). It is cemented into the under-surface of the acromium at its anterior end. It has been used infrequently and has allowed a modest gain in abduction with an unconstrained prosthesis in wholly rotator cuff-deficient patients. Loosening of the spacer or the glenoid component has not been encountered.

The second type of spacer was reported in 1982 by Clayton, Ferlic and Jeffers. A shaped block of high-density polyethylene was sutured to the undersurface of the coracoacromial ligament with four non-adsorbable sutures. This implant was designed for use with the Neer Mark II system but had not been used at the time it was reported. There are no subsequent reports of its use.

The third design was described by Grammont in *Surgery of the Shoulder* by Bateman and Welsh (1984). Called the Acropole prosthesis, it consisted of a curved hemiprosthesis screwed into the coracoid and bolted into the inferior

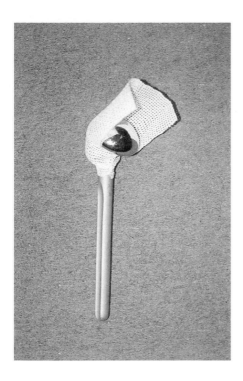

Figure 1.9 The Nottingham hood Mark IV prosthesis.

surface of the acromium in the line of the coracoacromial ligament. This articulated with a curved prosthetic insert in the form of a curved strip arching over the superior pole of the humeral head. Pain relief from this prosthesis was good, but gains in power and range of movement were poor, and it has not been widely used.

More recently, Wallace (1990) has designed a rotator cuff substitute for use with the Neer prosthesis in patients with an irreparable rotator cuff. A tube of Dacron is slipped over the humeral component before its insertion and pulled tightly around the prosthetic neck. The free edge is then trimmed to size and the remains of the rotator cuff are sutured to it. This accessory has afforded greater stability in the potentially unstable rotator cuff-deficient unconstrained shoulder but has not given the expected gains in power or range of movement (Figure 1.9).

Resection and interposition arthroplasty

In 1909, Rovsing injected sterile Vaseline into the shoulders of two patients. Both patients had excellent relief of pain, both at rest and on movement.

Interposition of a malleable material between arthritic joint surfaces has since been tried by several workers but, despite good early results, complications occur frequently, and the technique has not gained popularity.

Since 1952, Ivalon sponge, a vinyl plastic sponge, has been used for interposition arthroplasty and its use in two rheumatoid shoulders was reported in 1967 by Cobey. Both were said to have had excellent results although 'excellent' was not defined. Dislocation of the implant was said to have been prevented by fibrous ingrowth into the mesh of the prosthesis.

In 1980 Varian presented his results of 32 interposition arthroplasties using a silastic cup in 29 patients. Good pain relief was achieved and some gain in range of movement at the scapulothoracic joint was observed. No increase in glenohumeral movement was recorded. Five prostheses dislocated and four tore. In a subsequent paper by Spencer and Skirving (1986), six of 12 shoulders had a complication after follow-up of only 15 months; four had dislocated and two fragmented. A further patient had not had relief of pain. They concluded that this operation was only appropriate for rheumatoid patients whose humeral head remained hemispherical. Worries about silicone synovitis have dissuaded other workers from using this material.

In 1983, Thabe and Tillman reported the technique of resection interpositional arthroplasty in which a thorough synovectomy and subacromial bursectomy is combined with trimming of all osteophytes, excavation of all humeral and glenoid cysts and reduction in size and reshaping of the humeral head. Any remaining cysts are then bone grafted and the humeral head is covered with lyophilized dura. Koneczny (1986) reported the use of the same technique but used corium for covering the humeral head. Lyophilized dura was used by Miehlke, Thabe and Stegers (1987), who presented their results in 32 patients. Of these, 94% had benefited and were rated satisfactory, with all but five patients having good pain relief, and the average gain in elevation being 65°. Despite these encouraging results, the technique has not gained popularity.

The present

Despite the success of the Neer prosthesis and its worldwide acceptance as the most frequently used total shoulder arthroplasty, work continues to develop on an alternative which performs as well but involves removal of less bone and can be anchored without bone cement. In the USA Gristina and Webb have developed the 'monospherical' shoulder. Similar to the St Georg, it has a stemmed humeral ball of 40 or 44 mm diameter articulating with a metal-backed glenoid component supported on a trapezoidal keel, which is longer inferiorly to make best use of the cancellous bone towards the axillary border of the scapula. Warren and Dines of New York have developed the biomodular shoulder. Designed (but not yet licensed) for cementless fixation, the titanium stem has sintered beads around its collar and a cylindrical stem. A reversed Morse taper allows insertion of a choice of three humeral head sizes and three neck lengths. The glenoid is available in high-density polyethylene or metal backed with snap-in high-density polyethylene inserts. The metal-backed tray is secured by means of a central peg and two screws, a technique similar to that of the Post prostheses.

In the UK, Bayley has developed an unconstrained shoulder using a stemmed humeral component and an ovoid glenoid which is supported and secured by a self-tapping screw similar to that of the Kessel prosthesis. In Reading, Copeland has developed an unconstrained shoulder in which the humeral component is anchored into the humeral head without use of an intramedullary stem in the proximal humeral shaft and the pear-shaped glenoid was initially secured using a Freeman peg but his Mark II prosthesis has an uncemented glenoid peg (Figure 1.10).

In 1991 Wallace developed a prototype uncemented total shoulder arthroplasty which was further developed in 1994 as the Nottingham shoulder with porous ingrowth cobalt chrome surfaces on both glenoid and humeral components. Results of the use of these new prostheses have yet to be published but will be awaited with interest. No long-term results of any shoulder prosthesis have been reported and 10-, 15-, and 20-year follow-up of substantial numbers of patients is needed for a full evaluation. After years of experimentation it appears that a prosthesis which closely approx-

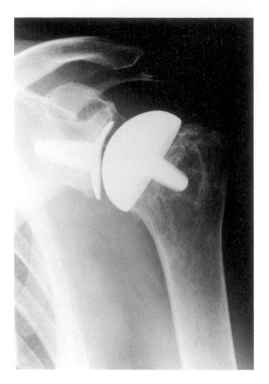

Figure 1.10 The Copeland Mark II prosthesis.

imates to the normal anatomy and which can be soundly secured in the severely eroded glenoid is most likely to be successful, provided that a sound rotator cuff reconstruction can also be achieved.

References

Albee FH (1921) Restoration of shoulder function in cases of loss of head and upper portion of humerus. *Surgery, Gynecology and Obstetrics* **32–1** 1–19.

Amstutz HC, Sew Hoy AL and Clarke IC (1981) UCLA anatomic total shoulder arthroplasty. *Clinical Orthopaedics and Related Research* **155** 7–20.

Bayley I and Kessel L (eds) (1982) The Kessel total shoulder replacement. In *Shoulder Surgery*, pp. 160–164. Berlin: Springer.

Beddow FH and Elloy MA (1977) The Liverpool total replacement for the gleno-humeral joint. In *Joint Replacement in the Upper Limb*, pp. 21–25. London: Institution of Mechanical Engineers.

Beddow FH and Elloy MA (1982) Clinical experience with the Liverpool shoulder replacement. In *Shoulder Surgery* (I Bayley and L Kessel, eds), pp. 164–167. Berlin: Springer.

Buechel FF, Pappas MJ and DePalma AF (1978) 'Floating-Socket' total shoulder replacement: anatomical, biomechanical and surgical rationale. *Journal of Biomedical*

Materials Research **129** 89–114.

Casuccio C (1966) Internal prostheses of the upper limb. *SICOT, 10th Congress of the International Society for Orthopaedic Surgery and Traumatology* (Paris), p. 62.

Clarke IC, Sew Hoy AL, Cruen TA and Amstutz HC (1981) Clinical and Radiographic assessment of a non-constrained total shoulder. *International Orthopaedics (SICOT)* **5** 1–8.

Clayton ML, Ferlic DC and Jeffers PD (1982) Prosthetic arthroplasties of the shoulder. *Clinical Orthopaedics and Related Research* **164** 184–191.

Cobey MC (1967) Arthroplasties using compressed Ivalon sponge. *Clinical Orthopaedics and Related Research* **54** 139–144.

Cofield RH and Stauffer RN (1977) The Bickel glenohumeral arthroplasty. In *Joint Replacements in the Upper Limb*, pp. 15–19. London: Institution of Mechanical Engineers.

Coughlin MJ, Morris JM and West WF (1979) The semiconstrained total shoulder arthroplasty. *Journal of Bone and Joint Surgery* **61A** 574–581.

Ducci L (1963) Sostituzione endoprotesica di estesa lisione omerale in granulomatosi eosinofila atipica. *Rivista degli Infortuni e delle Malattie Professionali* **51** 1236–1253.

Edelmann G (1951) Traitment immédiate des fractures complexes de l'extrémité de l'humerus par prothèse acrylique. *Presse Médicale* **59** 1777–1778.

Englebrecht E (1984) Ten years of experience with unconstrained shoulder replacement. In *Surgery of the Shoulder* (JE Bateman and RP Welsh, eds), pp. 234–239. St Louis: CV Mosby.

Englebrecht E and Stellbrink G (1975) Total shoulder replacement – design St Georg – preliminary report. *Scandinavian Journal of Rheumatology* **4** (Suppl. 8).

Fenlin JM (1975) Total glenohumeral joint replacement. *Orthopedic Clinics of North America* **6** 565–583.

Grammont PM (1984) The Acropole prosthesis. In *Surgery of the Shoulder* (JE Bateman and RP Welsh, eds), pp. 200–201. St Louis: Mosby.

Gristina AG and Webb LX (1982) The Trispherical total shoulder replacement. In *Shoulder Surgery* (I Bayley and L Kessel, eds), pp. 153–157. Berlin: Springer.

Haraldsson S (1969) Reconstruction of proximal humerus by muscle-sling prosthesis. *Acta Orthopaedica Scandinavica* **40** 225–233.

Jobbins B, Flowers M and Reeves BF (1973) Fixation of orthopaedic implants under tensile loading. *Biomedical Engineering* **Sept.** 380–383.

Jones L (1933) Reconstructive operation for non-reducible fractures of the head of the humerus. *Annals of Surgery* **97** 217–225.

Kenmore PI, Maccartee C and Brantley V (1974) A simple shoulder replacement. *Journal of Biomedical Materials Research* **5** 329–330.

Kessel L and Bayley I (1979) Prosthetic replacement of shoulder joint: preliminary communication. *Journal of the Royal Society of Medicine* **72** 748–752.

Kölbel R. (1984) Stabilization of shoulders with bone and muscle defects using joint replacement implants. In *Surgery of the Shoulder* (JE Bateman and RP Welsh, eds), pp. 281–293. St Louis: Mosby

Kölbel R and Friedebold G (1975) Schultergelenkersatz. *Zeitschrift für Orthopadie und ihre Grenzgebiete,* **113** 452–454.

Kölbel R, Rohlmann A and Bergmann G (1982) Biomechanical considerations in the design of a semiconstrained total shoulder replacement. In *Shoulder Surgery* (I Bayley and L Kessel, eds), pp. 144–152. Berlin: Springer.

Koneczny O (1986) *Die Koriumplastik in der Gelenk- und Extremitatenchirurgie.* Stuttgart: Thieme.

Krueger FJ (1951) A vitallium replica arthroplasty on the shoulder. *Surgery* **30** 1005–1011.

Lettin AWF (1982) Taking stock – ten years experience of shoulder arthroplasty. In *Shoulder Surgery* (I Bayley and L Kessel, eds), pp. 168–170. Berlin: Springer.

Lettin AWF and Scales JT (1972) Total replacement of the shoulder joint. *Proceedings of the Royal Society of Medicine* **65** 373–374.

Lettin AWF, Copeland SA and Scales JT (1982) The Stanmore total shoulder replacement. *Journal of Bone and Joint Surgery* **64B** 47–51.

Lugli T (1978) Artificial shoulder joint of Péan (1893). *Clinical Orthopaedics and Related Research* **133** 215–218.

Lynn TA, Alexakis PG and Bechtol CO (1965) Stem prosthesis to replace lost proximal humerus. *Clinical Orthopaedics and Related Research* **43** 245–247.

Macnab I (1977) Total shoulder replacement – a bipolar glenohumeral prosthesis. *Journal of Bone and Joint Surgery* **59B** 257.

Macnab I and English E (1976) Development of a glenohumeral arthroplasty for the severely destroyed shoulder joint. *Journal of Bone and Joint Surgery* **58B** 137.

Mathys R and Mathys R Jun. (1977) Isoelastische prothesen des schultergelenkes. *Aktuelle Probleme in Chirurgie und Orthopädie* **1** 9–16.

Miehlke RK, Thabe H and Stegers M (1987) Resection interposition arthroplasty of the rheumatoid shoulder. In *The Shoulder*. Proceedings of the 3rd International Conference on Surgery of the Shoulder (N. Takagishi, ed.), pp. 346–348. Tokyo: Professional Postgraduate Services.

Neer CS (1955) Indications for replacement of the proximal humeral articulation. *American Journal of Surgery* **89** 901–907.

Neer CS (1974) Replacement arthroplasty for glenohumeral osteoarthritis. *Journal of Bone and Joint Surgery* **56A** 1–13.

Neer CS (1984) Unconstrained shoulder arthroplasty. In *Surgery of the Shoulder* (JE Bateman and RP Welsh, eds), pp. 240–245. St Louis: Mosby.

Neer CS, Brown TH and McLaughlin HL (1953) Fracture of the neck of the humerus with dislocation of the head fragment. *American Journal of Surgery* **85** 252–258.

Neer CS, Watson KC and Stanton FJ (1982) Recent

experience in total shoulder replacement. *Journal of Bone and Joint Surgery* **64A** 319–337.

Péan JE (1894) Des moyens prothétiques destinés à obtenir la réparation de parties osseuses. *Gazette de Hôpitals Civils et Militaire (Paris)* **67** 291. (Republished in English translation: On prosthetic methods intended to repair bone fragments. *Clinical Orthopaedics and Related Research* **94** 4–7.)

Post M and Jablon M (1983) Constrained total shoulder arthoplasty. *Clinical Orthopaedics and Related Research* **173**, 109–116.

Post M, Haskell SS and Jablon M (1980) Total shoulder replacement with a constrained prosthesis. *Journal of Bone and Joint Surgery* **62A** 327–335.

Post M, Jablon M, Miller H and Singh M (1979) Constrained total shoulder joint replacement: a critical review. *Clinical Orthopaedics and Related Research* **144** 135–150.

Reeves B, Jobbins B and Flowers M (1972) Biomechanical problems in the development of a total shoulder endoprosthesis. *Journal of Bone and Joint Surgery* **54B** 193.

Reeves B, Jobbins B, Dowson D and Wright V (1971) The development of a total shoulder joint endo-prosthesis. *Conference on Human Locomotor Engineering*, pp. 69–75. London: Institution of Mechanical Engineers.

Reeves B, Jobbins B, Dowson D and Wright V (1972a) A total shoulder endo-prosthesis. *Engineering in Medicine* **1** 64–67.

Reeves B, Jobbins B, Flowers M, Dowson D and Wright V (1972b) Some problems in the development of a total shoulder endo-prosthesis. *Annals of the Rheumatic Diseases* **31** 425–426.

Richard A, Judet R and René L (1952) Reconstruction prothétique acrylique de l'extrémité supérieure de l'humérus spécialement au cours des fractures-luxations. *Journal de Chirurgie* **68** 537–547.

Rovsing T (1909) Treatment of dry arthritis with injection of Vaseline. *Annals of Surgery* **50** 1052–1076.

Rovsing T (1910) El tilfaelde af fri knogletransplantation til erstatning of overamens overste to trediedele ved hjaelp af patientens fibula. *Hospitalstidende* **53** 7–17.

Siegel A and Engelbrecht E (1977) Schultergelenkendoprothese 'St Georg'. *Aktuelle Probleme in Chirurgie und Orthöpadie* **1** 64–65.

Siegel A, Buchholz HW, Engelbrecht E and Rottger J (1977) The non-blocked shoulder endo-prosthesis. In *Joint Replacement in the Upper Limb*, pp. 27–31. London: Mechanical Engineering Publications, Institution of Mechanical Engineers.

Skillern PG (1920) Sarcoma of the humerus: resection of the upper shaft of the humerus with transplantation of the upper third of the fibula to the humerus stump. *International Clinics* **1** 41–44.

Spencer R and Skirving AP (1986) Silastic interposition arthroplasty of the shoulder. *Journal of Bone and Joint Surgery* **68B** 375–377.

Swanson AB (1984) Bipolar inplant shoulder arthroplasty. In *Surgery of the Shoulder* (JE Bateman and RP Welsh, eds), pp. 211–223. St Louis: Mosby.

Thabe H and Tillmann K (1983) Spatergebnisse von resektionsarthroplastiken der oberen extremitat bei chronischer polayarthritis im vergleich zur allo-arthroplastick. *Orthopädisch Praxis* **9** 662.

van der Ghinst M and Houssa R (1951) Acrylic prosthesis in fractures of the head of the humerus. *Acta Chirurgica Belgica* **50** 31–40.

Varian PW (1980) Interposition Silastic cup arthroplasty of the shoulder. *Journal of Bone and Joint Surgery* **62B** 116–117.

Wallace WA (1990) The Nottingham Dacron hood reinforcement for unconstrained shoulder replacement. In *Surgery of the Shoulder* (M Post, BF Morrey and RJ Hawkins (eds), pp. 277–281. St Louis: Mosby–Year Book.

Welsh RP and Macnab I (1985a) Arthroplasty of the shoulder. In *Practical Shoulder Surgery* (M Watson, ed.), pp. 40–41. London: Grune and Stratton.

Welsh RP and Macnab I (1985b) Arthroplasty of the shoulder. In *Practical Shoulder Surgery* (M Watson, ed.), pp. 52–53. London: Grune and Stratton.

Wheble VH, Skorecki J and Thompson G (1977) The design of a metal-to-metal total shoulder joint prosthesis. In *Joint Replacement in the Upper Limb*. pp. 7–13. London: Institution of Mechanical Engineers.

Zippel J (1975) Luxationssichere schulterendoprosthese modell BME. *Zeitschrift für Orthopadie und ihre Grenzgebiete* **113**, 454–457.

2

Shoulder movements and the biomechanics of the shoulder

W. Angus Wallace

The main function of the shoulder is to position the hand for activities of daily living, work and sports. The shoulder is not one individual joint but a complex of joints which allow the upper limb to be stabilized in a wide variety of positions of function without pain and with good strength. To do this a number of unique biomechanical characteristics come into play, both with regard to the movements or kinematics of the shoulder and relating to the forces involved in shoulder movement – the kinetics of the shoulder. Before concentrating on these, the anatomy of the shoulder will be reviewed, focusing on the areas of most interest with regard to joint replacement.

Anatomy of the shoulder region

The shoulder complex includes the scapula and clavicle, which form the pectoral girdle, providing a stable support for the glenoid, which articulates with the humeral head (Figure 2.1). When the upper limb moves, so also does the pectoral girdle, with movements taking place in five separate areas:

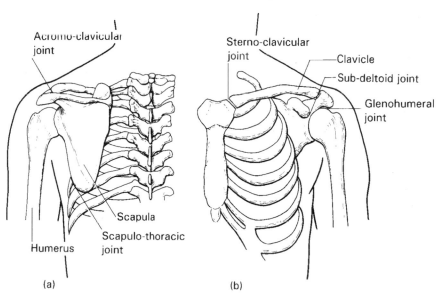

Figure 2.1 The joints of the shoulder complex, looking (a) from the back and (b) from the front.

1 At the sternoclavicular joint – whenever the scapula moves the sternoclavicular joint also undergoes some degree of movement.
2 At the acromioclavicular joint – this joint is stabilized primarily by the coracoclavicular ligaments, which allow movement to occur between the clavicle and the scapula.
3 At the scapulothoracic joint – this is a 'muscle sliding' joint which allows the scapula, anchored to the chest through the serratus anterior muscle attached along its medial border, to slide over the underlying rib cage, with the main movement occurring in the loose areolar tissue that lies between the serratus anterior muscle and the chest wall.
4 At the glenohumeral joint – although accepted as the main shoulder articulation, this joint is only responsible for two-thirds of the movement that occurs at the shoulder.
5 At the subacromial joint – this joint is worthy of a separate description because it is the site of the majority of shoulder symptoms, forming a structure very similar to a joint, with a roof (formed by the acromion posteriorly and the coracoacromial ligament anteriorly), a floor (formed by the supraspinatus tendon and the greater tuberosity inferiorly) and a joint cavity (formed by the subacromial bursa) which allows a free sliding movement between the floor below and the roof above (Figure 2.2).

Subacromial joint

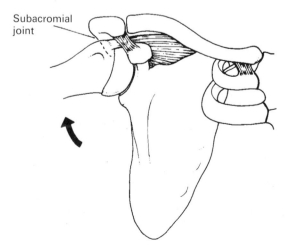

Figure 2.2 The subacromial joint – the location of the majority of shoulder pain.

Shape of the glenoid and humerus

The glenoid is almost oval with the appearance of an inverted comma and normally its long (vertical) axis lies almost parallel to the medial border of the scapula. Its transverse axis lies in a plane which is retroverted at an average of 7° to the blade of the scapula (Saha, 1973), but the exact angle of retroversion is difficult to establish because it changes, moving from the superior pole of the glenoid down to the inferior pole (Figure 2.3). The size of the articular surface of the glenoid is variable but on average measures 45 × 32 mm in the British population.

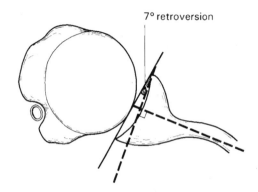

7° retroversion

Figure 2.3 The glenoid is usually retroverted (mean = 7°) with respect to the body of the scapula but this changes from the top to the bottom of the glenoid.

For many years the humeral head has been considered to lie in line with the humeral shaft, retroverted at an angle of 30–40° to the transepicondylar line of the elbow (Morrey and An, 1990). Research by Roberts et al (1991) has demonstrated that the humeral head is retroverted only 27° relative to the elbow *but* the centre of the humeral head is offset approximately 5 mm posteriorly from the line of the humeral shaft. This is shown in Figure 2.4, which demonstrates how the offset significantly alters the shape of the proximal humerus. The articular surface of the humeral head is very close to being spherical, with a mean diameter of 50.3 mm (CI, 49.6 to 51.1 mm) as reported by Roberts et al (1991).

Mobility of the shoulder

The most mobile segment of the shoulder complex is normally the glenohumeral joint

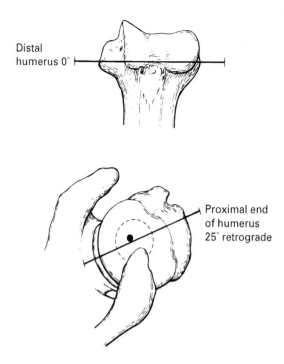

Distal humerus 0°

Proximal end
of humerus
25° retrograde

Figure 2.4 The humeral head has been shown to be only 21° retroverted with respect to the elbow but the centre of the head is 5 mm posteriorly offset with respect to the humeral shaft (Roberts et al, 1991).

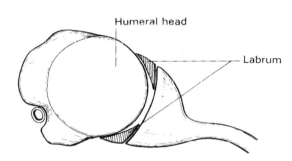

Humeral head

Labrum

Figure 2.5 The glenoid is considerably deepened by the glenoid labrum (shown viewed from above).

which allows a remarkable range of movement of the humerus on the scapula. The humeral head articulates with the glenoid face which is flatter than the head and only one-third of its surface area (Kent, 1971). The contact area between the glenoid and the humeral head is increased and improved by the presence of a fibrous labrum attached around the bony rim of the glenoid which functions in a similar fashion to the meniscus in the knee (Figure 2.5). It has been shown that the labrum improves the

humeral fit to the glenoid, with a mean vertical index (humeral head diameter/glenoid diameter) of 75% in a vertical analysis and 56% in a transverse analysis (Saha, 1973). The main benefit from this is the improved stability that occurs in the glenohumeral joint because of the consequent deepening of the socket, which has clearly been demonstrated by Lippitt et al (1993). An additional effect is the vacuum or suction effect which has been demonstrated to occur when the glenoid labrum 'sticks on to' the humeral head during attempted distraction of the humeral head from the glenoid (Lazarus et al, 1996).

When the glenohumeral joint is altered by arthritis or fracture there is often a reduction of movement at this joint, but a compensatory increase in movement at other joints. For arthritic patients this is most commonly appreciated as an increased strain placed upon the acromioclavicular joint giving rise to acromioclavicular joint pain – a well-recognized problem in patients with rheumatoid arthritis (Kelly, 1992).

Resting alignment of the shoulder

In the healthy shoulder, when the subject stands with the upper limb hanging down, the pectoral girdle adopts a remarkably constant position. The scapula lies at an angle of approximately 30° or 40° to the coronal plane, thus accommodating the 27° retroversion of the humeral head as shown in Figure 2.6a. The face of the glenoid lies with a downward tilt of approximately 5° compared with the vertical (Freedman and Munro, 1966; Walker, 1977; Wallace, 1982).

In the arthritic or stiff shoulder, and particularly with rheumatoid arthritis affecting the shoulder, the position of the scapula on the chest wall changes in response to the disease process. The scapula frequently becomes retracted, pulled posteriorly around the chest wall, coming to lie closer to the coronal plane – at an angle of 10° or 20° to the coronal plane. In association with the backward retraction of the scapula, the clavicle also angles anterosuperiorly, changing from its normal position of 5–10° of upward tilt to an upward angulation of 20–30° to the horizontal (Figure 2.6b). This abnormal positioning of the scapula is either due to contracture of some of the scapular

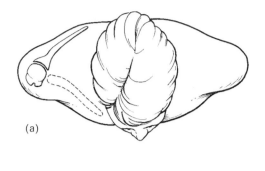

(a)

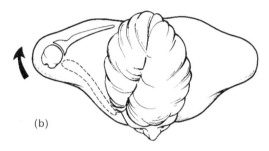

(b)

Figure 2.6 (a) The normal position of the scapula at rest. (b) The typical deformity in patients with rheumatoid arthritis.

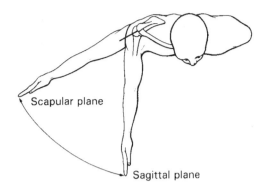

Figure 2.7 The plane of 'elevation' is variable and lies between the scapular and the sagittal planes.

stabilizing muscles or it may be a compensatory repositioning of the scapula to allow for more functional movements of the upper limb in the presence of a stiff glenohumeral joint.

Movements or kinematics of the shoulder

The main movements at the shoulder are elevation, internal and external rotation and horizontal flexion and extension. Although abduction in the plane of the scapula is the usual movement reported in scientific studies of the shoulder, this movement is generally not a valuable functional movement.

Elevation

Elevation is a much more functional movement of the shoulder and may occur in any plane between abduction in the scapular plane and forward flexion (Figure 2.7). For practical purposes it is the plane in which the arm can be lifted to its highest position while standing or sitting and is recorded as the angle between the upper arm or humerus and a vertical line passing through the shoulder joint. Normal

ranges of elevation starting with the arm dependant (i.e. at 0°) have been reported as a mean of 167° for men and 171° for women (Freedman and Munro, 1966; Doody, Freedman and Waterland, 1970). Elevation is one of the movements which is lost in the arthritic patient and it is often not possible for the rheumatoid patient to lift the arm above 60°.

Normal scapulohumeral rhythm

During elevation of the normal arm (or abduction in the scapular plane) there is a smooth movement of the scapula, which moves in concert with the movement of the glenohumeral joint. This coordinated action is described as normal scapulohumeral rhythm and only occurs when the glenohumeral joint is free of disease and the muscles around the shoulder are functioning normally. Although early static studies on scapulohumeral rhythm had indicated that there might be a more complicated relationship between scapular rotation and glenohumeral movement (Poppen and Walker, 1976), later dynamic studies have confirmed that, in most individuals, scapulohumeral rhythm is smooth throughout most of elevation, with a ratio of 2° of glenohumeral movement for every 1° of scapular rotation, as shown in Figure 2.8 (Wallace, 1982). Some researchers have endeavoured to separate the elevation that occurs at the glenohumeral joint (glenohumeral elevation) and that which occurs at the scapula (scapular rotation), but accurate and repeatable measurements of these two movements in normal clinical practice are virtually impossible. It has become the

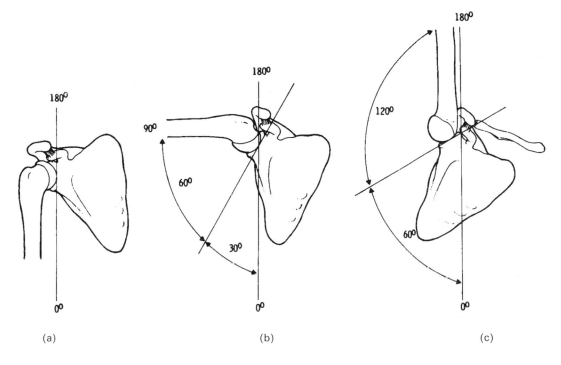

Figure 2.8 Scapulohumeral rhythm – smooth movements in a ratio of 2 : 1 of glenohumeral : scapular rotation during elevation.

author's practice to record only the movement of combined elevation using a fluid-filled goniometer.

Abnormal and reversed scapulohumeral rhythm

When the normal smooth coordinated movement between the scapula and the glenohumeral joint is lost, the scapulohumeral rhythm becomes abnormal. This is a clinical diagnosis based on simple observation, from the back, of the shoulders during elevation or abduction of the shoulders while the subject is standing.

Often the subject will be seen to 'hitch' the shoulder during elevation or suddenly the glenohumeral joint stops moving with more of the movement occurring at the scapula for part of elevation. If the glenohumeral joint is stiff and the range of glenohumeral movement is *less than* the range of scapular rotation, the scapulohumeral rhythm is said to be reversed.

Rotation of the shoulder during elevation

As the arm is raised, the humerus automatically externally rotates (Figure 2.9) to allow the whole of the articular surface of the humeral

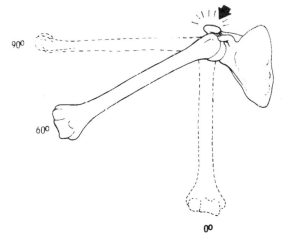

Figure 2.9 External rotation of the humerus occurs automatically as the arm is elevated, partly to avoid impingement of the greater tuberosity.

head to be used for joint movement and also to allow the greater tuberosity of the humerus to escape from beneath the coracoacromial arch, where it would impinge if rotation did not occur. This mechanical requirement is highlighted in the clinical situation, after shoulder replacement, when a patient with an internal

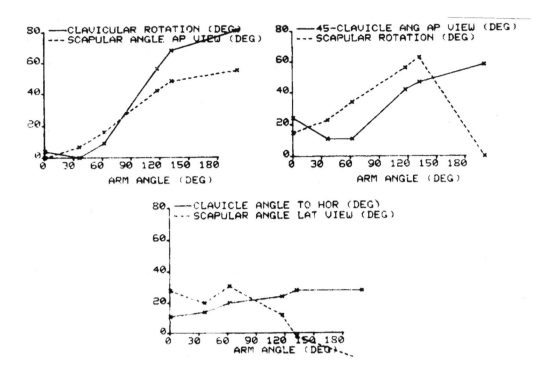

Figure 2.10 The graphs show the relative movements of the clavicle and scapula during arm elevation. Clavicle rotation along its axis is compared with scapular rotation as seen in the anteroposterior (AP) view. Clavicle angulation as seen in the 45° oblique view is associated with scapular rotation and the clavicular angle to the horizontal is compared with scapular angulation as shown in the lateral view. Where the lines diverge, acromioclavicular joint movement is occurring.

rotation contracture does not have the tight muscles released at operation. The result is that elevation will be limited owing to the impingement which occurs and the shoulder may become painful on attempted elevation above shoulder level.

Vertical displacement of the humeral head

Displacement of the humeral head on the glenoid during arm movement is an important component of shoulder movement during elevation and abduction. Poppen and Walker (1976) have shown on static studies that the humeral head moves superiorly by about 3 mm during the first 60° of elevation and then remains fairly constant, with only 1 mm or at most 2 mm of movement upwards or downwards on the face of the glenoid. However, Wallace (1982) in dynamic studies has shown that the humeral head starts off with its centre 1–2 mm higher than the midpoint of the glenoid; the head then moves upwards by about 3 mm during the first 90° of elevation and

thereafter slides down and laterally on the glenoid to a position 2–3 mm below the midpoint of the articular surface of the glenoid. Clearly this upward movement may result in impingement of the supraspinatus tendon under the coracoacromial arch occurring in the shoulder. After shoulder replacement in a patient who has 'rotator cuff deficiency' this upward migration of the humeral head can be observed and pain is often reported by the patient.

Active and passive rotation of the shoulder

Although much emphasis has been placed on shoulder elevation, perhaps the most disabling form of shoulder stiffness is loss of rotational movements. Experience with patients who have had shoulder arthrodeses confirms that after glenohumeral joint fusion the range of shoulder rotation is reduced to a maximum range of 20–30° of total rotation. This highlights the fact that the normal 70° of external (lateral) rotation and 90° of internal (medial) rotation is predominantly a glenohumeral joint movement. It is therefore not surprising that when the glenohumeral joint becomes arthritic this rotational movement is the first to be lost. In general most individuals do not notice loss of rotational movement until their internal rotation is reduced to below 50° and their external rotation range is down to less than 30°. In the rheumatoid shoulder loss of external rotation is particularly bothersome. This occurs partly as a result of subscapularis contracture, but also because of the tendency of the scapula to move posteriorly around the chest wall.

Movements of the acromioclavicular joint

When the arm is raised the scapula moves on the chest wall, but the movements of the scapula and the clavicle, although linked, are not identical. This means that during elevation there is movement at the acromioclavicular joint, which is only minimal below 90° of arm elevation but then increases steadily up to full elevation, as shown in Figure 2.10 (Wallace and Johnson, 1982).

Forces involved in shoulder movement – kinetics of the shoulder

The forces required to elevate the arm are much larger than commonly appreciated. Figure 2.11 shows the lever arm lengths for the upper limb. For a 70 kg man the moment required to balance an arm held at 90° of abduction is 1.16 kg.ms when there is no weight in the hand, but this is increased to 2.43 kg.ms when a 2 kg weight is held in the hand. For the deltoid alone to sustain this position a force of 43 kg (with a 28 mm lever arm) would be required for the unladen arm but that force would be increased to 87 kg (greater than body weight) when holding a 2 kg weight. Poppen and Walker (1978) developed a mathematical model to explore the likely forces occurring around the shoulder and commented that using only a 1 kg weight in the hand would increase the loads in the deltoid and supraspinatus by over 60%. Similar findings were reported by Wallace (1984) when a cadaveric shoulder and arm specimen was actively loaded using cables to reproduce the forces generated by both the deltoid and the supraspinatus muscles. The results for an arm held in 30, 60 and 90° of

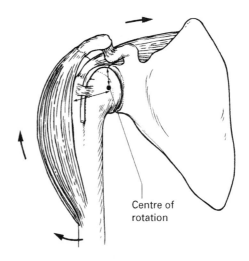

Figure 2.11 Forces occurring in the shoulder joint.

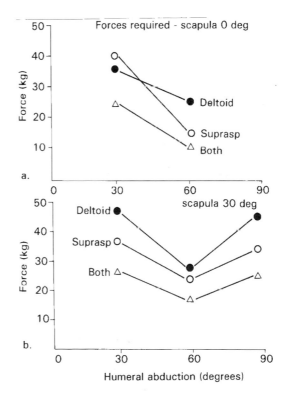

Figure 2.12 Forces in the deltoid and supraspinatus muscles: (a) scapula at 0°; (b) scapula at 30°. ●, Deltoid; ○, supraspinatus; △, both. (Wallace, 1982).

abduction (taking into account the normal scapular rotation) are shown in Figure 2.12. These findings emphasize the large forces transmitted across the glenohumeral joint which equate to 1× body weight with the arm unladen and 2–3× body weight when loads are held in the outstreched arm. In addition, Poppen and Walker (1978) have shown that there is a shear force of 0.42× body weight acting upwards on the glenoid when the arm is held in 60° of abduction.

Muscles acting on the glenohumeral joint

The muscles around the true shoulder joint can be divided into two main groups: the movers and the humeral head stabilizers.

The *movers* are:

- The deltoid, divided into three parts: the anterior third with unipennate fibres which flexes and internally rotates; the powerful middle third with multipennate fibres which abducts; and the posterior third with unipennate fibres which extends and externally rotates.
- The latissimus dorsi which adducts, extends and internally rotates, but which acts directly between the trunk and the proximal humerus.
- The pectoralis major which adducts, flexes (up to 90°) and internally rotates and also acts directly between the trunk and the proximal humerus.
- The teres major which adducts, internally rotates and extends.

The *humeral head stabilizers* include all the rotator cuff muscles and the long head of the biceps muscle:

- The supraspinatus, which also acts as an ancillary abductor.
- The infraspinatus, which is also the primary external rotator.
- The subscapularis, which also acts as an ancillary internal rotator.
- The teres minor, which both pulls down the humeral head and adducts the shoulder.
- The long head of the biceps, which depresses the humeral head when the arm is in external rotation and resists anterior subluxation when the head is in internal rotation, in addition to its function as an elbow flexor.

The function of the movers is easy to understand from the origins and insertions of the

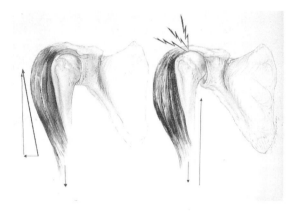

Figure 2.13 Humeral head impingement from the unopposed action of the deltoid.

respective muscles. The function of the humeral head stabilizers is, however, much more complex. If the deltoid contracts alone, the effect is to force the humeral head upwards, and pain is caused when the humeral head squeezes (or impinges) the rotator cuff between the humeral head below and the coracoacromial arch above (Figure 2.13). It is therefore essential to stabilize the humeral head and hold it downwards and centrally on the glenoid. The capsule of the shoulder and the rotator cuff muscles normally do this, in addition to other mechanisms including the coraco-humeral ligament.

Stabilization of the humeral head

Stabilization of the humeral head is produced by five main mechanisms:

1 The subscapularis–infraspinatus–teres minor (SIT) sling mechanism.
2 The supraspinatus and long head of biceps bowstring mechanism.
3 Gravity acting on the arm, tending to depress the humeral head.
4 Internal negative pressure within the shoulder joint cavity.
5 The capsular restraining ligaments (in particular the coracohumeral ligament).

Subscapularis–infraspinatus–teres minor (SIT) sling

The rotator cuff supporting the humeral head can be likened to a sling. The deltoid produces a strong upward force, while the tendinous cuff

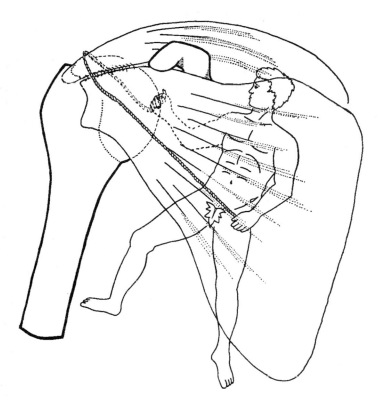

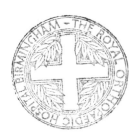

Figure 2.14 The lower fibres of subscapularis anteriorly and the infraspinatus and teres minor posteriorly pull the humeral head down using the supraspinatus tendon as a sling. A longitudinal tear in the supraspinatus tendon will interfere with this mechanism.

produces a compensatory downward pull (Figure 2.14). The muscles actively producing this downward pull are the subscapularis in front and the infraspinatus and teres minor behind. The sling is completed by the apical tendinous part of the cuff which is formed by the tendinous portion of the supraspinatus. The stabilizing effect of the SIT sling will be lost if there is a longitudinal tear of the supraspinatus tendon or a widening of the rotator interval. The rotator interval is the fibrous junction of the subscapularis and supraspinatus tendon, which usually blends closely or fuses close to the cuff attachment to the greater tuberosity of the humerus.

Supraspinatus and long head of biceps bowstring mechanism

Both the supraspinatus and the long head of biceps tendon arch over the curved surface of the humeral head. Because both are deformed by the humeral head and because both tendons are taut during certain shoulder movements, they produce a stabilizing resultant force which helps maintain the humeral head centrally on the glenoid (Figure 2.15). To be effective, the bowstring effect of the supraspinatus can only occur if other forces are used to stabilize the greater tuberosity.

Gravity effects on the arm

The weight of the upper limb is approximately 5.2% of body weight, or equivalent to 3.6 kg for the average 70 kg man. When standing, this weight tends to counteract the upward pull of the deltoid muscle.

Internal negative pressure within the shoulder

The concept of stabilization of the shoulder by negative pressure was recognized by Codman in 1934 but this mechanism has only been investigated and proved to be effective since the 1980s. Helmig et al (1992) and Wülker,

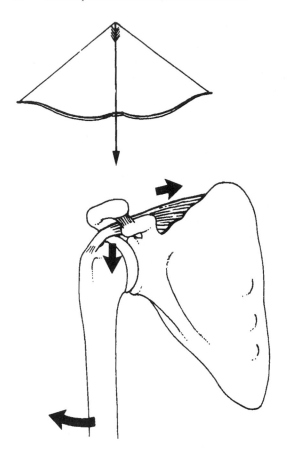

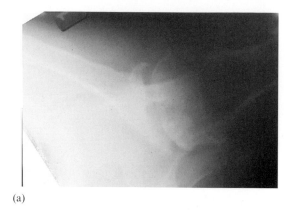

(a)

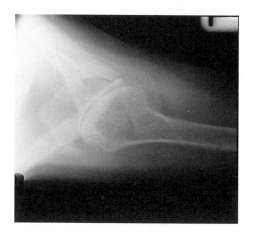

(b)

Figure 2.15 The bowstring mechanism used by the suppraspinatus to stabilize the humeral head.

Figure 2.16 (a) and (b) The posterior bony loss and consequent retroversion of the glenoid commonly seen in osteoarthritis.

Sperveslage and Brewe (1992) have reported their observations in cadavers and confirmed that the negative pressure inside the joint may be responsible for up to 50% of its overall stability.

Capsular restraining ligaments

DePalma et al (DePalma, 1973; DePalma, Callery and Bennett, 1980) and Gagey et al (1987) have described the coracohumeral and glenohumeral ligaments as checkreins which become taut and prevent humeral head displacement in certain positions. More recently Clark and Harryman (1992) have reviewed the anatomy of the glenohumeral ligaments and have stated that the exact function of all the ligaments in the region of the shoulder has yet to be clarified and that further mechanical testing is required.

Changes in glenohumeral shape in disease

Osteoarthritis usually produces a loss of bone from the posterior half of the glenoid, resulting in an increase in apparent retroversion of the glenoid (Figure 2.16). The author believes this may be secondary to the contracture of the anterior capsule which often accompanies the arthritis. However, sometimes the tightness is the primary cause of the arthritis, as is seen after an excessively tight Putti–Platt operation for recurrent anterior dislocation.

In rheumatoid arthritis the shoulder suffers bony damage to both sides of the joint, with medialization of the glenohumeral joint due to significant glenoid erosion and bone loss (Figure 2.17a). As the humeral head moves

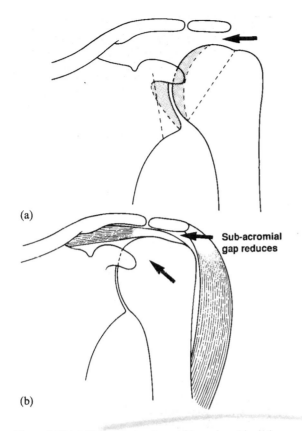

(a)

Sub-acromial gap reduces

(b)

Figure 2.17 (a) The typical pattern of bone loss (shaded area) seen in rheumatoid arthritis. (b) The typical medial and upward migration which occurs in rheumatoid arthritis. Note this radiological appearance usually indicates an intact rotator cuff.

medially, it also moves upwards and there is a reduction in the acromiohumeral distance, as shown in Figure 2.17b. The result is a secondary entrapment of the humeral head under the acromion and limitation of gleno-humeral movement. At the time of shoulder arthroplasty, the surgeon needs to take this problem into account by relocating the humeral head well below the acromion and as far laterally as possible. The appropriate surgical techniques are dealt with in detail in Chapter 7.

Changes in the rotator cuff in disease

In osteoarthritis of the shoulder the rotator cuff is usually unaffected, with healthy tendons and no rotator cuff tear unless the disease is secondary osteoarthritis due to rotator cuff pathology. In rheumatoid arthritis it has always been assumed that rotator cuff tears are common but it has been the experience of both the author, in a consecutive series of 40 shoulder replacements, and of Kelly (1994) that less than one-fifth of patients with rheumatoid arthritis undergoing shoulder arthroplasty have full-thickness tears, although 30% have thin rotator cuff tendons which must be treated with respect at the time of surgery (Kelly, 1994).

References

Basmajain JV and Blatant FG (1959) Factors preventing downward dislocation of the adducted shoulder – an electromyographic study. *Journal of Bone and Joint Surgery* **41A** 1182–1186.

Clark JM and Harryman DT II (1992) Tendons, ligaments and capsule of the rotator cuff. *Journal of Bone and Joint Surgery* **74A** 713–725.

Codman EA (1934) *The Shoulder*. Boston: Thomas Todd. (Republished by Robert E. Krieger Publishing Company, Florida, 1984.)

DePalma AF (1973) *Surgery of the Shoulder*, 2nd edn, pp. 206–210, 229. Philadelphia: Lippincott.

DePalma AF, Callery G and Bennett GA (1980) Shoulder joint. 1. Variational anatomy and degenerative lesions of the shoulder joint. In *Instructional Course Lectures, The American Academy of Orthopaedic Surgeons* **6** 255–281.

Doody SG, Freedman L and Waterland JC (1970) Shoulder movements during abduction in the scapular plane. *Archives of Physical Medicine and Rehabilitation* **51** 595–604.

Freedman L and Munro R (1966) Abduction of the arm in the scapular plane: scapular and gleno-humeral movements. *Journal of Bone and Joint Surgery* **48A** 1503–1510.

Gagey O, Bonfait H, Gillot C, Hureau J and Mazas F (1987) Anatomic basis of ligamentous control of elevation of the shoulder (reference position of the shoulder joint). *Surgical and Radiological Anatomy* **9** 19 26.

Helmig P, Suder P, Sojbjerg JO and Ostgard SE (1992) Glenohumeral instability following puncture of the joint capsule: an experimental study. *Journal of Bone and Joint Surgery* **74B** (Suppl.) 10–11.

Kelly IG (1992) The source of shoulder pain in rheumatoid arthritis. Its implications for surgery. *Journal of Shoulder and Elbow Surgery* (in press).

Kelly IG (1994) Unconstrained shoulder arthroplast in rheumatoid arthritis. *Clinical Orthopaedics* **307** 94–102.

Kent BE (1971) Functional anatomy of the shoulder complex. *Physical Therapy* **51** 947.

Lazarus MD, Sidles JA, Harryman DT, Matsen FA (1996) Effect of a chondral-labral on glenoid concavity and geno-humeral stability. A cardaveric model. *Journal of Bone and Joint Surgery* (A) **78A** 94–102.

Lippitt SB, Vanderhooft JE, Harris SL, Sidles JA, Harryman DT II and Matsen FA (1993) Glenohumeral stability from concavity-compression: a quantitative analysis. *Journal of Shoulder and Elbow Surgery* **2** 27–35.

Morrey BF and An K-N (1990) Biomechanics of the shoulder. In *The Shoulder* (CA Rockwood and FA Matsen, eds) pp. 208–245. Philadelphia: Saunders.

Poppen NK and Walker PS (1976) Normal and abnormal motion of the shoulder. *Journal of Bone and Joint Surgery* **58A** 195–201.

Poppen NK & Walker PS (1978) Forces and the glenohumeral joint in abduction. *Clinical Orthopaedics* **135** 165–170.

Roberts SNJ, Foley APJ, Swallow HM, Wallace WA and Coughlan DP (1991) The geometry of the humeral head and humeral prosthesis design. *Journal of Bone and Joint Surgery* **73B** 647–650.

Saha AK (1973) Mechanics of elevation of glenohumeral joint. *Acta Orthopaedica Scandinavica* **44** 668–678.

Walker PS (1977) *Human Joints and their Artificial Replacements*. Springfield, IL: Thomas.

Wallace WA (1982) The dynamic study of shoulder movement. In *Shoulder Surgery* (I Bayley and L Kessel, eds), pp. 139–143. Berlin: Springer.

Wallace WA (1984) Evaluation of the forces, ICR and the neutral point during abduction of the shoulder. *Transactions of the 30th Annual Meeting of the Orthopaedic Research Society* **9** 5.

Wallace WA and Johnson F (1982) A biomechanical appraisal of the acromioclavicular joint. In *Shoulder Surgery* (I Bayley and L Kessel, eds), pp. 179–182. Berlin: Springer.

Wülker N, Sperveslage C and Brewe F (1982) The contributions of capsule and atmospheric pressure to glenohumeral joint stability. A biomechanical study. Poster presented at the *5th International Conference on Surgery of the Shoulder* (Paris, July 1992).

3

Indications for shoulder replacement and shoulder assessment

Christopher R. Constant

As with all forms of surgery, the final result inevitably depends on good patient selection for the procedure. This is particularly so in shoulder replacement. A clear understanding of the indications for surgery, together with realistic expectations by doctor and patient, will give satisfying results. On the other hand, the indiscriminate use of shoulder replacement, without careful preoperative patient selection, will give rise to unsatisfactory results and unhappy patients.

In considering the indications for shoulder replacement, it is important not only to know the absolute indications for surgery but also to be aware of the limitations of the procedure in individual patients. While obvious clinical indications for shoulder replacement may be present, other over-riding considerations may well make the surgery inappropriate. Prior to surgery, it is important to consider such matters as the patient's general health, the condition of other joints, particularly in the upper limb, the need to use walking aids, as is often the case in rheumatoid arthritis, as well as the patient's general expectations of what can be achieved. The patient must have a clear knowledge of what can be realistically accomplished. Clearly if the patient's expectations are unrealistic, then success in terms of achieving the patient's objective is unlikely.

It is therefore important that the preoperative selection process be undertaken carefully, and should consist of establishing not only the presence of a clinical disorder for which shoulder replacement may be appropriate but also the suitability of the patient for the procedure.

Therefore, in considering the indications for shoulder replacement, one must look at the clinical indications, the objectives of surgery and how these may affect the clinical indications, and overall patient selection in relation to physical disease, mental attitude towards the procedure and its results, and the patient's motivation towards undertaking often difficult, prolonged and complex rehabilitation following such surgery. On the other hand, it may be that the indication for surgery is pure pain relief, without improvement in other aspects of shoulder function, and in this situation the patient must be truly aware of what the surgery is all about.

In discussing shoulder assessment, Constant and Murley (1987) noted the importance of distinguishing between the diagnostic and functional shoulder assessments undertaken before surgery, the former being that assessment used to establish a diagnosis for which shoulder replacement may be appropriate, and the latter to establish the degree of functional disability present before surgery, and subsequently after surgery to assess progress resulting from the procedure.

Clinical indications

In the 40 years since the publication in 1955 of Neer's original work on articular head replacement for fractures of the shoulder, the indica-

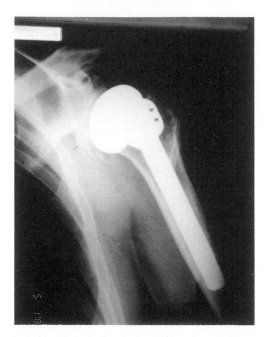

Figure 3.1 Hemi-shoulder arthroplasty.

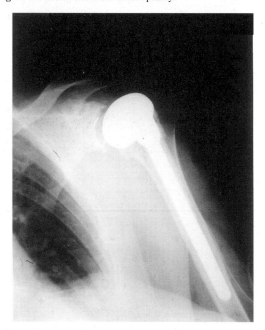

Figure 3.2 Total shoulder arthroplasty.

tions for hemiarthroplasty (Figure 3.1) and total shoulder arthroplasty (Figure 3.2) have become more clearly defined. The original indication for the use of shoulder replacement at that time was for proximal humeral fractures, where avascular necrosis of the humeral head was an expected complication. The indications now include fractures, rheumatoid arthritis, osteoarthrosis in all its forms, whether primary or secondary, and avascular necrosis. Shoulder replacement is now also indicated in some instances after tumour excision, where custom-built prostheses may be used.

'Functional' versus 'limited goal' surgery

Before considering the individual clinical indications for the procedure, it is worth remembering that the goal of surgery should be clearly defined. This may be divided into either a 'functional' objective or a 'limited goal' objective. In a functional objective, there should be a predetermined goal towards which the patient should aspire. This usually includes pain relief and a particular painless functional range of active movement with which the patient can then use the shoulder in normal everyday activities. It is frequently possible to predict the functional goal of shoulder replacement in different clinical conditions, but the final achievement after surgery is highly dependent on the patient's own motivation to undertake and persist with the extensive prolonged physiotherapy and exercise programme. Failure to partake of this rehabilitation may well preclude achieving a predetermined goal. It is therefore important to establish the patient's motivation before surgery, but it is not always possible to do so. Many patients are well motivated and this becomes clear on initial interview and subsequent interviews and examinations. It is also often apparent from the outset that patients are not prepared to undertake the rehabilitation programme, and in such circumstances it should be made clear to them that the functional success may not be great. There is a group of patients in whom it is difficult to assess motivation on the basis of one or more interviews. In such situations, the clinical and functional assessment should be combined with an assessment by the physio-therapist, who can often pick up the frequently subtle signs of the patient's intention to co-operate or not. Unfortunately, in some circumstances, preoperative motivation appears good but disappears postoperatively, leaving the patient with a satisfactory operative and radiological result but little in the way of functional improvement apart from pain relief. Great care, and indeed considerable time, is sometimes necessary to determine the patient's motivation in circumstances where this is in some doubt at the time of initial interview and examination. In cases of four-part fractures, with or without dislocations, where a hemiarthroplasty is considered, the time constraints upon proceeding with the operation sometimes make it difficult to assess patients' motivation; the results of such surgery can be variable, although, on the whole, if patients are reasonably selected on first and possibly second interview, the results are very encouraging.

In general terms, if one looks at the clinical indications for shoulder replacement, assuming good motivation on the part of the patient, it is apparent that the final result of shoulder replacement frequently depends on the condition of the neighbouring soft tissues, particularly the rotator cuff and its reconstruction at the time of surgery, if this is feasible. One can therefore perhaps simply divide the indications for shoulder replacement into those in which a functionally good result can be expected, and those in which pain relief is the prime objective. In patients with osteoarthrosis, excluding rotator cuff arthropathy, avascular necrosis and four-part fracture, one could expect a good functional result with worthwhile active motion and pain relief. This could also apply to rheumatoid arthritis if the rotator cuff is still intact and functioning. In many cases of rheumatoid arthritis the rotator cuff is incompetent, whether torn or not, and this usually results in a somewhat limited postoperative active range of motion, but pain relief can be very dramatic.

Therefore, along with the true clinical indications, there should be a comment as to whether one can reasonably expect a functional result or a limited goal result. As will be seen later the author considers that, the assessment of function includes assessment of pain severity, and therefore pain relief of itself does improve function. Similarly, the relief of pain for activities of daily living undertaken in a limited way can make such activities more effective, and this must also be considered when looking at the indications for shoulder replacement.

Osteoarthrosis

Hip and knee replacement surgery are well-established procedures undertaken by the ma-

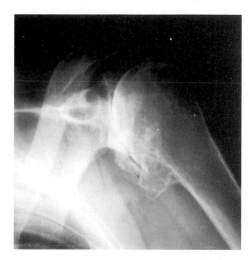

Figure 3.3 Primary osteoarthritis of the shoulder.

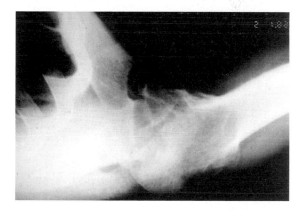

Figure 3.4 Secondary arthrosis caused by trauma.

jority of general orthopaedic surgeons, with reasonable results expected. Primary osteoarthrosis of the shoulder (Figure 3.3) is a less common condition but is now no less amenable to replacement than other joints. As is discussed elsewhere in this text, the technical procedure of shoulder replacement differs from that of the hip in that the reconstruction of the soft tissues is of paramount importance in achieving a good result. The presence of symptomatic osteoarthrosis in a well-motivated patient is a clear indication for shoulder replacement, which in this situation can be expected to give excellent results. The decision as to whether to use a hemi- or total shoulder replacement remains open to discussion, and various series have attested to the good results from both procedures in appropriate cases.

Secondary osteoarthrosis (Figure 3.4) as a result of previous trauma is a good indication for functional replacement. The end result does depend on the nature of the previous trauma, particularly in relation to what damage occurred to the soft tissues. Pain relief, and often a more functional objective, can be expected after shoulder replacement in these circumstances.

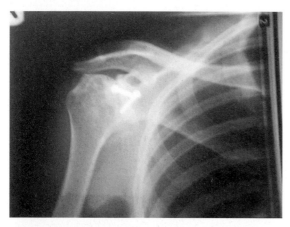

(a)

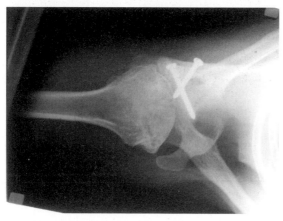

(b)

Figure 3.5 Osteoarthosis secondary to previous surgery for posterior instability. (a) Anteroposterior view. (b) Axial view.

Osteoarthrosis after previous surgery, often for recurrent dislocation, is frequently associated with shortening of the soft tissues, anteriorly or posteriorly, depending on the procedures previously undertaken. Figure 3.5 shows the radiographs of a 40-year-old female patient who underwent a posterior bone block and posterior muscle shortening procedure at the age of 15 years for recurrent posterior instability. The functional end result of surgery

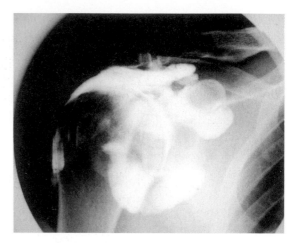

Figure 3.6 Shoulder arthrogram showing a torn rotator cuff and flow of contrast into the acromioclavicular joint – Geiser sign.

in these circumstances may well depend on the ability to lengthen, mobilize and reconstruct the rotator cuff at the time of surgery, and failure to undertake such a reconstruction may present one with a limited goal-type surgery. Careful preoperative assessment of the soft tissues, with radiographs, an arthrogram (Figure 3.6), computerized tomography (Figure 3.7) and magnetic resonance imaging (Figures 3.8 and 3.9), may well help in establishing a reasonable postoperative objective. Pain relief is usually good.

The specific form of osteoarthrosis known as rotator cuff arthropathy (Figure 3.10), in which there is global absence of the rotator cuff and the humeral head subluxes upwards, ultimately to articulate on the undersurface of the acromion (with or without erosion of the acromion or acromioclavicular joint), is difficult to treat satisfactorily. Rockwood (1989) described good results from debridement of the humeral head and subacromial space, and the author's limited experience with this procedure has produced good results. The use of a large-head hemi- or total arthroplasty or the use of a constrained arthroplasty may be considered in this situation. In the majority of such cases, surgery can only be expected to give a limited goal result, with pain relief and passive motion and an improvement of overall function as a result of these. The inevitable complication of loosening after insertion of a constrained shoulder prosthesis should always be kept in mind when considering this surgery. The absence of satisfactory soft tissues is a relative

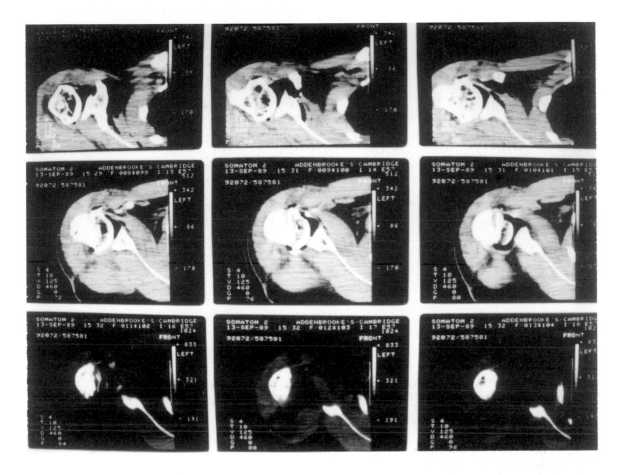

Figure 3.7 Computerized tomogram of shoulder, showing a displaced humeral head fracture.

contraindication to shoulder replacement (see Contraindications p. 37).

Rheumatoid arthritis

There is a large spectrum of severity in rheumatoid arthritis, ranging from the mild to moderate disease (Figure 3.11), with an intact and indeed functioning rotator cuff, to severe erosive de-structive arthropathy (Figure 3.12), with little or no bone left in the region of the proximal humerus and significant loss of soft tissue cover. Ranging from one extreme to another is the possibility of achieving a good result on the one hand, and an unsatisfactory result, even for pain relief, on the other. In rheumatoid arthritis the primary indication for shoulder replacement is pain. In the presence of reasonable soft tissue cover, and less than total

destruction of the humeral head, in the presence of reasonable bone stock, one can expect moderate functional return after shoulder replacement. In the presence of a well-preserved glenoid, hemi-shoulder arthroplasty can give as good results as total shoulder arthroplasty. In the presence of total destruction of the shoulder joint, it is unrealistic to expect more than pain relief. Considering rheumatoid arthritis as an indication for shoulder replacement, it is important to assess function in the other joints. It is of considerable importance to establish the function in the lower limbs in patients who need to use walking aids. It is the author's experience that the use of a walking aid after shoulder replacement frequently gives rise to further pain, despite early reasonable results in respect of pain relief. Similarly it is important to consider the other joints in the upper limb, especially the elbow. The overall function of the

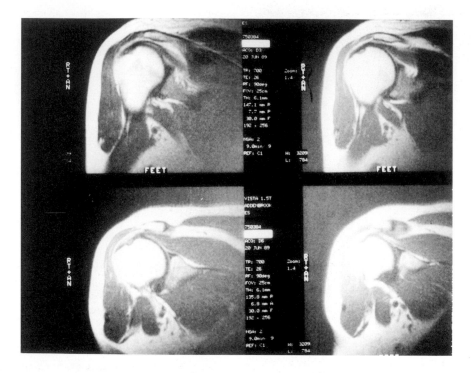

Figure 3.8 Magnetic resonance scan, showing the subacromial area.

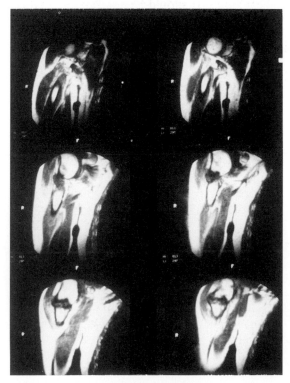

Figure 3.9 Magnetic resonance scan showing humeral head and surgical neck fracture which is ununited.

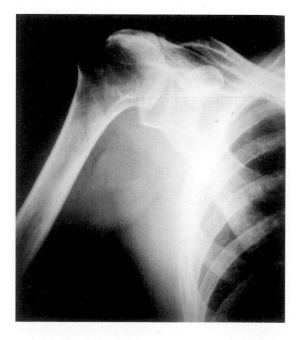

Figure 3.10 Radiograph showing rotator cuff arthropathy.

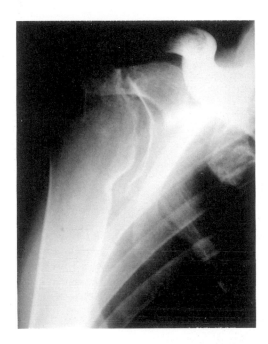

Figure 3.11 Moderate rheumatoid arthritis.

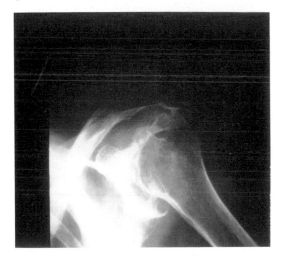

Figure 3.12 Severe late rheumatoid arthritis.

upper limb is a combination of shoulder, elbow, wrist and hand function, and if elbow and distal arm function is significantly impaired, then a reasonable shoulder can help in a limited way to improve things, but obviously cannot be expected to overcome some of the disabilities related to the more distal joints.

Finally, in considering rheumatoid arthritis and shoulder replacement, it may be necessary to consider a shoulder replacement merely to improve passive shoulder rotation in order to provide a safe basis for proceeding with an elbow replacement. An essential prerequisite for a successful elbow replacement is a reasonably mobile shoulder. In the presence of a stiff shoulder, aseptic loosening of an elbow replacement is inevitable, and it may therefore be necessary to precede elbow replacement with a shoulder replacement, merely to achieve passively mobile shoulders, to avoid such complications after elbow surgery.

Avascular necrosis

Avascular necrosis (Figure 3.13) affecting the humeral head usually results from the long-term use of steroids or from radiotherapy for Hodgkin's disease or breast cancer. It may also result from trauma, particularly a fracture of the anatomical neck (Figure 3.14), with or without associated fractures of the surgical neck and tuberosities. In these circumstances, if the glenoid is well preserved, as indeed it often is, then a hemiarthroplasty (Figure 3.16) can be expected to give good results in the well-motivated patient, and return the shoulder to near normal. It should be remembered that the soft tissues around the shoulder may be grossly constricted after radiotherapy, and extensive soft tissue dissection may be necessary in order

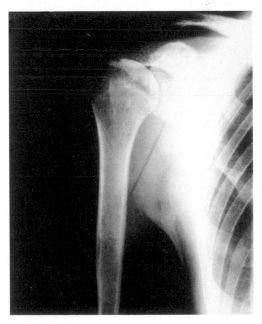

Figure 3.13 Early avascular changes in a patient on long-term steroid therapy for ulcerative colitis.

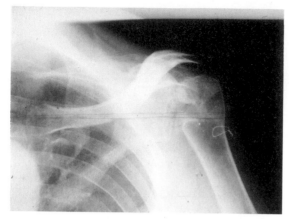

Figure 3.14 Old four-part proximal humeral fracture with humeral head necrosis.

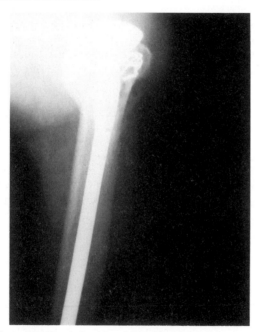

Figure 3.15 Hemi-shoulder arthroplasty inserted for a four-part fracture with wiring of the tuberosities.

to achieve a satisfactory soft tissue lengthening and reconstruction. This in turn may present problems in relation to the brachial plexus and neurovascular bundle, which may well be densely adherent to the underlying subscapularis and may present difficulties, in terms of both bleeding and neuropraxiae, during mobilization of this muscle. In considering avascular necrosis following radiotherapy, this fact should be remembered and appropriate discussion with the patient about these complications and their likely results should be undertaken before surgery is performed.

Trauma

The pre-eminent indication in trauma is the four-part fracture dislocation of the proximal humerus in an elderly patient (Figure 3.16). Primary humeral head replacement in these circumstances can be expected to give excellent functional results. The author now routinely uses the excised humeral head as a subtuberosity bone graft in this procedure, assisting early union of the tuberosities to the humeral shaft. An intensive early postoperative rehabilitation programme is thus possible, and with good patient co-operation a near normal shoulder function can be expected. Obviously a clear prerequisite for a good result is good patient motivation. In the elderly group in which this injury occurs, motivation is frequently lacking; the results of surgery may well prove to be disappointing in these patients. As previously mentioned, it is often difficult to assess patient motivation on the basis of one interview after the fracture has been sustained. If, however, the patient is reasonably *compos mentis*, accepts the pro-cedure and is prepared to consider the postoperative rehabilitation, then four-part fracture dislocation in the elderly is a realistic indication for primary humeral head replace-

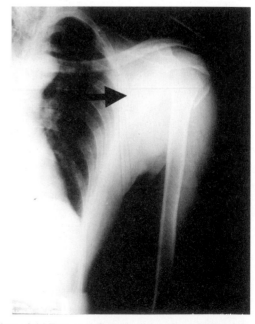

Figure 3.16 Four-part fracture dislocation of the proximal humerus. The arrow shows the dislocated head fragment.

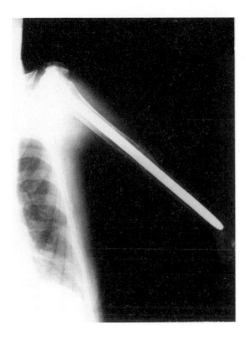

Figure 3.17 Long-stem hemiarthroplasty used to achieve union of a humeral shaft fracture in a patient with a stiff rheumatoid shoulder proximal to the fracture.

ment. Such a procedure would not be indicated in the presence of severe dementia.

Debate continues as to whether the three-part fracture, or the four-part fracture in the younger age group, constitutes an indication for shoulder replacement. Gerber (1989) reported good functional results after multiple wiring for comminuted fractures of the upper limb. Careful consideration in planning shoulder replacement is also required in a situation where a patient suffers a fracture of the proximal shaft of the humerus in the presence of a stiff shoulder or of rheumatoid arthritis. It is difficult to get such fractures to unite, particularly in the elderly patient. The use of a hemiarthroplasty to achieve a mobile shoulder and early union of the fracture, using the excised humeral head as a bone graft, can achieve excellent results in these patients (Figure 3.17), and may return a patient to independence, whereas continuing disability from an ununited fracture and stiff shoulder may well prevent such a return.

Contraindications

In the author's opinion, the only absolute contraindication to a shoulder replacement is evidence of continuing infection. As in other joints, the insertion of a prosthesis into an infected site is a disaster. A relative contra-indication to shoulder joint replacement is severe soft tissue incompetence. Absence of deltoid function, global rotator cuff absence or any condition in which deltoid or rotator cuff function is severely impaired should be carefully considered when assessing the indications for shoulder replacement. In these situations the use of a constrained arthroplasty may prove necessary in order to achieve stability in the flail shoulder. In a situation where pain is a particular problem such an operation may be appropriate. In the absence of pain it is often difficult to justify such a procedure, on the basis of the known incidence of loosening of such constrained prostheses. A large-head arthroplasty, acting as a subacromial spacer, may well improve function a little, and may have to be considered in such circumstances. Mention has already been made of the problems of rotator cuff arthropathy, in which there is a global absence of the rotator cuff, where the difficulties encountered are similar to those being discussed here.

It is therefore apparent that pure clinical or radiological indications for shoulder replacement exist but must always be combined with an appropriate assessment of the patient's motivation and expectations of the surgery.

Assessment

The author believes that the assessment of the shoulder should be divided into a diagnostic and a functional assessment. The diagnostic assessment involves the history, physical examination and elicitation of specific physical signs, radiological and sometimes haematological investigation, and special investigations including contrast radiography, computerized tomography, magnetic resonance imaging and arthroscopy. Such a diagnostic investigation results in an anatomical, physiological and pathological diagnosis of the problems involved. Such assessment does not, however, give an indication of the level of function of an affected shoulder. It is therefore important to separate the functional assessment of the shoulder from the diagnostic assessment, although the parameters used for functional assessment are of course used in part of the diagnostic assessment.

Name :   Date :
Address   Number :
                                          Date of birth :
                                          .. / .. / ....

Occupation :   Rt. / Lt. handed

General health :

Past history :

Drugs/allergies :

Main symptoms :   pain/stiffness/weakness
                              right/left

Pain :   day/night   With :   activity/rest

At :   below waist/waist to shoulder/above shoulder height

Type of pain :   (1)   localized pain - site

                    (2)   diffuse deep pain

                    (3)   aching type pain - ? radiation

                    (4)   painful arc - ? range

Injury ?   yes/no

If yes :   date :
              details :

History of present complaint :

Treatment to date :

Limitations of activities of daily living :
              work :
              sport/hobbies :
              sleep :

? Pain on lying on the affected side :   yes/no

Figure 3.18 Constant Shoulder Diagnostic Assessment: history.

Stewart and Hundley (1955) and Hawkins and Hobeika (1983) described methods whereby an allocation of points for specific physical signs and investigative results was used in order to obtain a functional level. In theory it should be that, in this situation, the more points obtained (the more abnormal physical signs), the lower the functional ability of the shoulder. However, there is no evidence to suggest that there is an inverse ratio of any kind between the presence of physical signs and the level of shoulder function. Therefore the use of this method of assessment of shoulder function is unsuited to most forms of clinical work and clinical research into shoulder problems. Indeed, it is not uncommon for a paucity of signs

Name :   Number :   Date :

EXAMINATION

Neck :

General signs :

Contour :   right/left

Scapulothoracic rhythm :   normal/abnormal   right/left

Wasting (site) :   right/left

Tenderness (site) :   right/left

GLENOHUMERAL JOINT :   <u>Right</u>   <u>Left</u>

Flexion :   Active
                       Passive

Abduction :   Active
                       Passive

Internal rotation :   Active
                       Passive

External rotation :   Active
                       Passive

Glenohumeral crepitus :   yes/no   right/left

Painful arc :   yes/no   right/left
                       Angle of arc :   ... - ...   abduction
                                         ... - ...   flexion
                                            - ...   rotation

Power of abduction :   right :   left :

Instability :
Apprehension   +/-   right/left   external/internal rotation
Sulcus sign   +/-   right/left
Displacement   +/-   right/left   anterior/posterior

Figure 3.19 Constant Shoulder Diagnostic Assessment: neck, general and glenohumeral signs.

---

to be associated with severe functional disability. The converse of this statement is also true. An extreme example of such a paradox would be the paralysed shoulder, where signs may be few and perhaps include only wasting and paralysis, while function is of course severely disabled. In this situation a low diagnostic score, if such a score were to be used to decide

function, would result in a high functional score. In such a paralysis an extremely low functional score may be expected, in the presence of few physical signs. There must therefore remain a clear distinction between the diagnostic and functional assessments of the shoulder. In assessing functional progress after surgery, or in disease, the functional scoring

NAME :   NUMBER :   DATE :

SUBACROMIAL :

Tenderness :   right/left   Acromial edge/Supraspinatus

Impingement :   right/left   +/-

ACROMIOCLAVICULAR JOINT :	<u>Right</u>	<u>Left</u>
Type (contour) :	1/2/3	1/2/3
Tenderness :	+/-	+/-
Pain with horizontal compression :	+/-	+/-
Pain with vertical compression :	+/-	+/-
Instability : anterior / posterior	+/-	+/-
superior / inferior	+/-	+/-

STERNOCLAVICULAR JOINT :		
Swelling :	+/-	+/-
Tenderness :	+/-	+/-
Instability :	+/-	+/-

<u>Any other findings :</u>

<u>Plain radiographs :</u>   (../.../....)   RIGHT/LEFT

<u>Arthrogram :</u>   (../.../....)   single/double contrast   right/left

<u>Arthroscopy :</u>   (../.../....)

<u>Other investigations :</u>

Diagnosis :

Figure 3.20 Constant Shoulder Diagnostic Assessment: acromioclavicular and sternoclavicular joints and investigations.

---

is the relevant one. The diagnostic score, as mentioned, allows one to make a diagnosis, but the functional score defines the ability or disability of the shoulder regardless of such a diagnosis. While the physical signs, the diagnostic and investigative procedures and the continuing assessment of physical signs may be of great prognostic significance after treatment, and indeed must be of great diagnostic significance before surgery, they are frequently of little functional value to the patient or surgeon. It is also obvious that serological, haematological and radiological findings, although relevant to patient care, have little in the way of relevance to the patient's shoulder function, and therefore allocation of points to such parameters as radiographs, blood test results and physical findings like clicks and crepitus have no place in the functional assessment of the joint.

Diagnostic assessment

The diagnostic assessment must consist of a detailed history, physical examination and investigations, including imaging, serological and others, so that an anatomical, physiological and ultimately pathological diagnosis may be made in every case. The detailed history of symptoms and their characteristics often gives the assessor a very good idea of the probable diagnosis. The history will also point to where examination should concentrate. A general physical examination as well as a detailed physical examination of the neck and both shoulders should always be undertaken. Clinical examination of the shoulder should be carried out in an orderly fashion, always including an examination of the neck, as well as a brief examination of the whole upper limb and the general condition of the patient. The diagnostic assessment is completed by the use of appropriate blood tests, and more frequently by the use of plain and contrast radiography, computerized tomography, magnetic resonance imaging and arthroscopy in certain cases. The author's own diagnostic forms are seen in Figures 3.18–3.20. In a situation where shoulder arthroplasty is being considered, symptoms and signs such as pain, stiffness, weakness and wasting, as well as bone to bone crepitus, are of particular importance in the history and physical examination. The use of diagnostic arthroscopy to assess patient motivation is a useful technique in certain circumstances: the observation of recovery from a minor procedure such as arthroscopy may well give an indication of the patient's motivation, in the event of major surgery being considered, as well as providing valuable information about the condition of the joint and the rotator cuff.

Functional assessment

This forms a separate part of the assessment and allows one to assess the functional ability of the shoulder at any one time, during progress of the disorder, or after treatment such as shoulder replacement. It allows comparable evaluation of the improvement or deterioration in shoulder function following treatment. The use of a method of functional assessment which allows easy evaluation of shoulder function will also allow comparable evaluation of results in individual patients, before and after treatment, in groups of patients and from different centres. Constant and Murley (1987) developed a method of functional assessment which consisted of a 100-point score based on the assessment of a number of individual subjective and objective parameters. This assessment is undertaken in a clinical setting. Other authors have described the use of a 100-point scoring system for shoulder joint assessment which included diagnostic and radiological findings in the scoring system, thereby (in this author's view) nullifying the assessment of pure function. Kessel and Bayley (1979) have expressed the opinion that individual parameter assessment on an ongoing basis is the best way to evaluate function, but this does not allow easy study of functional progress. The use of questionnaires, as described by Lipscombe (1975), provides an entirely subjective assessment, and in one method used by Stewart and Hundley (1955) the parameters used in assessing function varied depending on the diagnosis. The author considers the 100-point scoring system, combined with the ability to assess individual parameters with numerical values, to be the best method of functional assessment of the shoulder and has now effectively used this method of functional assessment of the shoulder for the past 13 years. The parameters are chosen for their functional relevance, and include pain, normal activities of daily living, active painless functional range of motion in four planes, and shoulder power. Tables 3.1–3.3 show scoring for individual parameters, scoring for pain experienced during normal daily activities and scoring for activities of daily living in relation to work, recreation, sport and sleep, and to positioning of the hand in relation to the trunk. The first subjective parameter assesses the most severe degree of pain experienced during normal activities of daily living. Absence of pain scores 15 points, while the presence of severe pain scores zero points (Table 3.2). The other subjective parameter assessed is the ability of the individual to carry out daily activities in relation to work, recreation

Table 3.1 Scoring for individual parameters

Parameter	Score
Pain	15
Activities of daily living	20
Range of motion	40
Power	25
Total	100

Table 3.2 Scoring for pain

Pain	Score
None	15
Mild	10
Moderate	5
Severe	0

Table 3.3 Scoring for activities of daily living

	Score
Activity level	
Full work	4
Full recreation/sport	4
Unaffected sleep	2
Positioning	
Up to waist	2
Up to xiphoid	4
Up to neck	6
Up to top of head	8
Above head	10
Total for activities of daily living	20*

*Only one of the five positions is found in each patient. The maximum points attainable by a normal individual in this section of the assessment can be only 20 points.

Table 3.4 Scoring for forward and lateral elevation

Elevation (°)	Score
0–30	0
31–60	2
61–90	4
91–120	6
121–150	8
151–180	10

Table 3.5 Scoring for external rotation

Position	Score
Hand behind head with elbow held forward	2
Hand behind head with elbow held back	2
Hand on top of head with elbow held forward	2
Hand on top of head with elbow held back	2
Full elevation from on top of head	2
Total	10

Table 3.6 Scoring for internal rotation

Position	Points
Dorsum of hand to lateral thigh	0
Dorsum of hand to buttock	2
Dorsum of hand to lumbosacral junction	4
Dorsum of hand to waist (3rd lumbar vertebra)	6
Dorsum of hand to 12th dorsal vertebra	8
Dorsum of hand to interscapular region (DV 7)	10

and the ability to sleep (Table 3.3). The ability of the patient to perform everyday activities in terms of the position of the arm in relation to the trunk is also evaluated. Twenty points are allocated for normal activities of daily living. Ten points are based on the patient's subjective answers regarding ability to perform normal work and recreation and ability to sleep. The other 10 points are allocated to activities of daily living in relation to the patient's ability to perform tasks at a variety of levels, ranging from below the waist to above the head. It should be noted that this is not the assessment of pure motion but that of the ability to place the hand in various positions to work at different levels, as described. Thus a combination of movements making up a functional

range is being assessed. The objective assessment rates the patient on painless active motion in the planes of pure forward and lateral elevation, as well as composite functional internal and external rotation. Scoring for these functional active painless motion ranges is shown in Tables 3.4–3.6.

Shoulder power is included in the assessment, and is measured as abduction power to a maximum of 90° against resistance. With the use of a spring balance (Figure 3.21) or other device which measures resisted power of abduction in pounds or kilograms, shoulder power can be easily, repeatedly and accurately assessed, with a maximum of 25 points being achieved for a maximum of 25 or more pounds painless resisted abduction. To work in kilograms, a simple conversion factor of 2.2 can be used. An example of a completed shoulder functional assessment form, as used by the author, is shown in Table 3.7.

Table 3.7 Shoulder function in a 60-year-old man with osteoarthritis of the right shoulder and a normal left shoulder

	Right	(score)	Left	(score)
Pain	Moderate	5	None	15
Activities of daily living				
Work	Full	4	Full	4
Recreation	Nil	—	Full	4
Sleep	Poor	1	Unaffected	2
Position	Top of head	8	Above head	10
Range				
Abduction (°)	90	4	180	10
Flexion (°)	105	6	180	10
Internal rotation	L5	4	T12	8
External rotation	Limited	4	Full	10
Power	10 lb (4.5 kg)	10	20 lb (9 kg)	20
Total	Right	46%	Left	93%

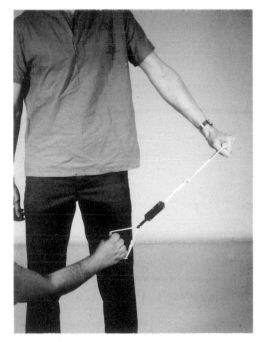

Figure 3.21 The use of a spring balance to test shoulder abduction power. The patient's maximum abduction was 40°.

Before undertaking shoulder replacement a careful diagnostic assessment will confirm the indications for such surgery, and a functional assessment will establish the degree of disability present. Repeated functional assessments at frequent intervals following surgery will allow easy determination of progress being made (whether improvement or deterioration) and, while providing a valuable aid to the surgeon in observing progress, it also provides excellent encouragement to patients to maintain their programme of rehabilitation in order to improve their function. With experience in the use of this method of shoulder assessment it is frequently possible to predict the degrees of functional ability that one can expect patients to recover after treatment for a variety of shoulder conditions.

Conclusion

In considering shoulder replacement, and its indications, the author is of the opinion that an important part of the assessment before surgery consists of a diagnostic assessment followed by a functional assessment. It is also important to have a clear indication of what the objective of surgery is. Before surgery, both the surgeon and patient should have a clear idea of the benefits to be gained, and in the absence of such information the question of shoulder replacement should be reconsidered. In the presence of appropriate indications, with proper patient selection and good motivation, one can expect reasonable progress after shoulder surgery, improvement of function with the passage of time and excellent results from the operation of shoulder replacement.

References

Constant CR and Murley AHG (1987) A clinical method of functional assessment of the shoulder. *Clinical Orthopaedics and Related Research* **214** 160–164.

Gerber C (1989) Multiple wiring of proximal humeral

fractures. In *Proceedings of the George Perkins Symposium* (London).

Hawkins RJ and Hobeika PE (1983) Impingement syndrome in the athletic shoulder. *Clinics in Sports Medicine* **2** 391–405.

Kessel L and Bayley I (1979) Prosthetic replacement of shoulder joint. *Journal of the Royal Society of Medicine* **72** 748–752.

Lipscombe AB (1975) Treatment of recurrent anterior dislocation and subluxation of the glenohumeral joint in athletes. *Clinical Orthopaedics and Related Research* **109** 122–125

Neer CS II (1955) Articular replacement for the humeral head. *Journal of Bone and Joint Surgery* **37A** 215–228.

Rockwood C, Gerber C and Wallace WA (1989) Debridement of massive rotator cuff tears. Personal communications.

Stewart MJ and Hundley JM (1955) Fractures of the humerus – a comparative study in methods of treatment. *Journal of Bone and Joint Surgery* **47A** 681–692.

4

Neer total shoulder replacement

Philip Hirst

There are many varieties of total shoulder replacement but they largely fall into two groups: those prostheses which are constrained, where stability is dependent upon the constraint of the articulation, and those that are relatively unconstrained, where stability and function are provided entirely by the soft tissues around the shoulder joint. It has long been known from studies of the hip, knee and indeed of early shoulder designs that constraint, whilst imparting stability, does lead to increased stresses at the bone–prosthesis junction and therefore to later loosening. This is well described by Lettin (Lettin, Copeland and Scales, 1982) who has reported a 20% loosening rate in his series using the Stanmore prosthesis.

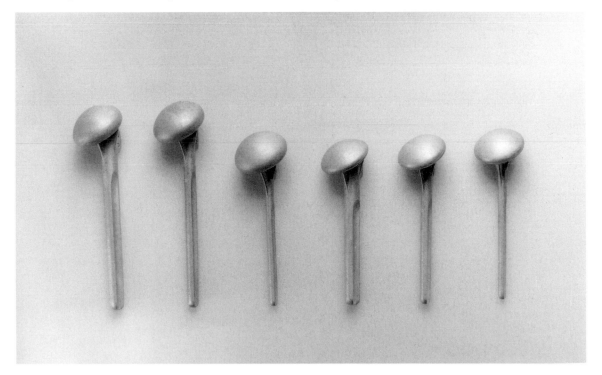

Figure 4.1 The six standard humeral components.

The function of any unconstrained prosthesis is dependent on the soft tissues, and in particular the rotator cuff. This inevitably means that the balance of the soft tissues and tensioning of the rotator cuff are critical if good results are to be obtained. If this goal of lack of constraint with soft tissue stability and good function can be achieved, then loosening ought to be a minor problem. Neer (Neer, Watson and Stanton, 1982) has shown the truth of this concept, and his prosthesis can provide excellent pain relief and function as well as standing the test of time in terms of component loosening.

Implant design

The humeral component (Figure 4.1) is made of cobalt chrome alloy and comes in two head thicknesses (22 and 15 mm) and three stem diameters (6.3, 9.5 and 12.7 mm). Extra-long and extra-short stem lengths are also available for particular cases. The radius of curvature of both head sizes is 44 mm and is designed to mimic the radius of the average humeral head. The glenoid component has a similar radius and is available either as a polyethylene or a metal-backed polyethylene prosthesis (Figure 4.2). The stem can be inserted either as a press-fit or with cement. It is important to cement the prosthesis when it is used for humeral fractures in order to control length and therefore soft tissue tension as well as controlling rotation. In the past, surgeons were divided in their opinion on the need for cement for the humeral component. But in the 1990s it became recognized that this design of humeral stem should be cemented. The glenoid component is designed specifically for insertion with cement.

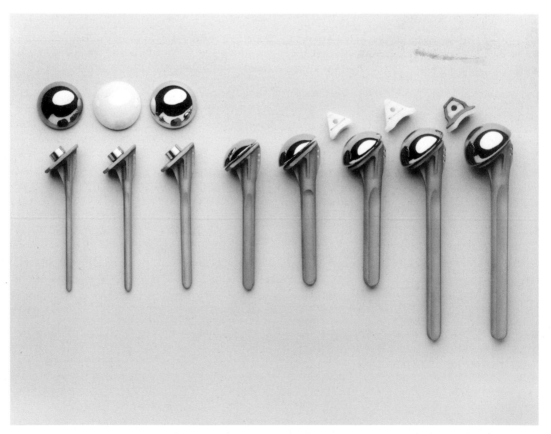

Figure 4.2 Metal-backed and polyethylene glenoid components. Wherever possible the metal-backed variety has been employed, although for small glenoids the polyethylene component, occasionally with the keel trimmed, has been used. (Courtesy of 3M Health Care Ltd.)

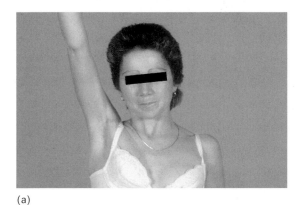

(a)

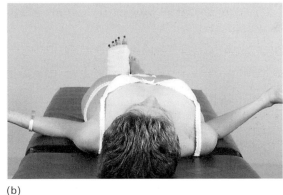

(b)

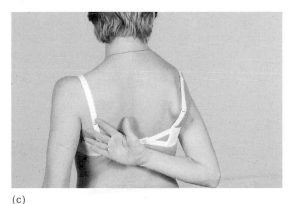

(c)

Figure 4.3 (a)–(c) A 34-year-old patient with rheumatoid arthritis, 2 years after a total shoulder replacement. She also had penicillamine-induced renal failure before her replacement, necessitating a successful renal transplant. She demonstrates virtually normal shoulder function.

Indications

Total shoulder replacement is primarily indicated for the relief of pain in those patients with a painful chronic glenohumeral incongruity. Although functional improvement is a welcome adjunct, we would not advise performing an arthroplasty solely to improve a poor range of movement in an otherwise painfree joint. It is surprising how some patients with a stiff shoulder and gross radiological destruction of the articular surface due to inflammatory joint disease can have a pain-free joint. These patients are not in general candidates for total shoulder replacement, unless pain becomes a significant symptom later.

The largest group of patients offered shoulder replacement suffer from an inflammatory polyarthropathy such as rheumatoid arthritis, seronegative arthritis or psoriatic arthropathy. Osteoarthritis of the shoulder is relatively uncommon but is a strong indication for total shoulder replacement. Avascular necrosis of the humeral head is rare but in general a humeral hemiarthroplasty only is indicated in these cases.

The age is not usually considered a problem as patients considered for shoulder replacement generally have multiple joint problems and the survival of the implant is probably greater in the shoulder than in the lower limb prostheses (Neer, Watson and Stanton, 1982). Our youngest patient, with rheumatoid arthritis, had her total shoulder replacement at the age of 32 and 2 years later had a fully functioning pain-free shoulder (Figure 4.3).

Contraindications to total shoulder replacement are recent local sepsis, paralysis of the deltoid and rotator cuff, and a neuropathic joint.

Important relative contraindications include the technical ability of the surgeon, the experience of the physiotherapist and the co-operation of the patient. The operation is a demanding one, and the best results are obtained by experienced surgeons working with skilled and experienced physiotherapists on well-motivated patients. The skill of the surgeon and the physiotherapist are of equal importance and for this reason total shoulder replacement should be performed in centres where there is a special interest in shoulder surgery. It is not an operation for the occasional surgeon.

Patient motivation is critical as the rehabilitation period is long and exacting, and the patient needs to understand that recovery is dependent, to a great extent, on his or her motivation and willingness to follow the postoperative regimen for many months.

Operative technique

As part of the preoperative work-up, the physiotherapist will discuss the postoperative regimen with patients so that they know what is expected of them.

All patients have an axillary shave on the day of operation, and the arm and upper chest are prepared with a topical alcoholic solution of povidone-iodine. Surgery is performed in an operating theatre equipped with a vertical laminar flow tent to reduce the chance of airborne infection. After induction of anaesthesia, 1500 mg cefuroxime is given by intravenous injection. This combination of clean air plus antibiotics should reduce the rate of infection dramatically (Lidwell et al, 1983) and Wallace (personal communication) has reported an infection rate of only 1 in 200 shoulder prosthesis operations using a similar regimen of prophylaxis.

The patient is positioned carefully on the table in a semisitting position. This reduces bleeding from the shoulder and provides for better access during surgery. It is essential that the patient is placed at the edge of the operating table to allow the arm to hang down freely. This will facilitate the reaming of the humerus. A small sandbag placed along the vertebral border of the ipsilateral scapula controls movement of the scapula during manipulation of the arm.

It is the policy on our unit to perform two skin preparations in a manner analogous to that used in the Centre for Hip Surgery at Wrightington hospital. The patient has the affected limb prepared and draped in the anaesthetic room after induction of anaesthesia, and a second preparation using povidone-iodine is performed in the operating theatre.

Surgical exposure

The surgical exposure of the shoulder used is

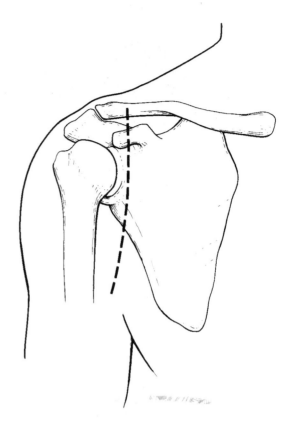

Figure 4.4 The skin incision for an extended anterior deltopectoral approach.

the extended anterior deltopectoral approach. The incision extends proximally from the acromioclavicular joint to the upper part of the arm (Figure 4.4). After the cephalic vein is identified, it is mobilized and retracted medically. Care should be taken to keep the vein intact, although if it is damaged no problems seem to arise from ligating it. The interval between deltoid and pectoralis major can now be developed and suitable retraction will expose the fascia overlying the coracoid muscles (Figure 4.5). At this point a finger should be introduced into the subdeltoid space to develop this space, and with care the deltoid can be separated completely from the upper humerus laterally from the posterior rotator cuff behind and from the superior rotator cuff on top.

The clavipectoral fascia is now split vertically, and the lateral edge of coracobrachialis identified. Blunt dissection with a finger will free both this muscle and the short head of biceps from the subscapularis muscle and the whole muscle mass can be retracted medially. In order to improve exposure further, either the

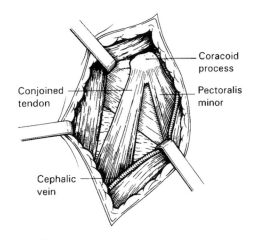

Figure 4.5 The deltopectoral groove opened, with the conjoined tendon and coracoid now visible.

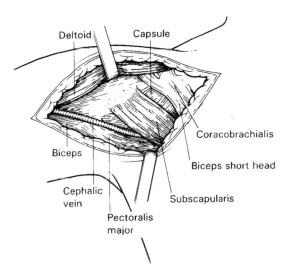

Figure 4.6 Lateral retraction on the deltoid with the arm abducted to 60° brings the subscapularis tendon and upper humerus into view.

upper part of the tendon of pectoralis major may be divided or the distal attachment of the anterior deltoid can be released. Just occasionally, in very difficult cases, even better access can be gained by releasing part of the conjoint tendon at the coracoid process as long as the majority of its fibres are left intact. Retraction in this area should always be gentle to avoid too much traction on the musculocutaneous nerve. Retraction of the deltoid laterally will provide a very satisfactory exposure of the subscapularis and the upper humerus (Figure 4.6).

Osteotomy of the clavicle (as described in

Chapter 7) greatly improves the exposure, and we have found it very valuable in dealing with complex fractures of the upper humerus but we have not found it necessary in a routine total shoulder replacement.

Neer (1988) has described division of the subscapularis tendon as the route into the joint. This may be necessary if there is an internal rotation contracture of the subscapularis as it will allow a Z-plasty to be performed to improve the external rotation. However, in those cases without a contracture, we prefer to perform an osteotomy of the lesser tuberosity and retract this structure medially with its attached subscapularis tendon. This gives an excellent exposure and the reattachment seems to be very strong, allowing early mobilization. To carry this out, the long head of biceps is first identified in its groove and an incision made along the rotator interval from the top end of the bicipital groove to the base of the coracoid process, thus mobilizing the upper border of the subscapularis. This incision is best made with the arm in full external rotation to lessen the risk of damage to the long head of biceps from the knife. The lower border of subscapularis is identified by the leash of blood vessels which accompany it. These may have to be ligated, and this is best done with the arm externally rotated to protect the axillary nerve. Two stay sutures of heavy absorbable material are placed in the tendon medial to the tuberosity. The lesser tuberosity is osteotomized using a large osteotome placed just medial to the biceps groove and directed towards the head, ensuring a good piece of bone is taken. The tuberosity can now be detached with the subscapularis and retracted medially and the muscle can be freed by blunt dissection from the front of the glenoid (Figure 4.7). Fibres will be found attaching it to the coracoid process and these should be divided.

The joint is now open, and further exposure is obtained by dividing the humeral head. The level of cut is a matter of judgement and it is always better to take too little rather than too much. It can be adjusted later. A prosthetic stem placed anterior to the upper humerus will act as a guide to the angle of the osteotomy. It is very important to prepare the humeral head in 30–40° of retroversion and this is best achieved by externally rotating the arm by 30° and then placing the prosthesis with its articular surface facing medially (Figure 4.8).

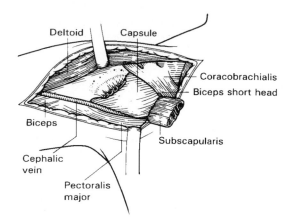

Figure 4.7 Either the lesser tuberosity is detached and retracted medially or the subscapularis is divided (as shown), exposing the shoulder joint.

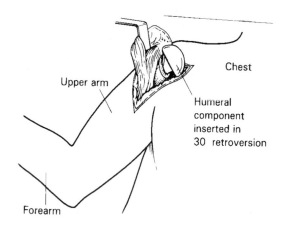

Figure 4.8 Position of patient, surgeon and arm in 30° external rotation (with respect to the surgeon) before osteotomizing the humeral head.

The rotator cuff can now be assessed and we recommend surgical repair of any tears at this stage. The techniques used do not differ from those required to repair rotator cuff tears in general (Neviaser and Neviaser, 1985), although massive tears will pose very difficult problems.

Mobilization of the rotator cuff

The posterior cuff can now be mobilized from the posterior rim of the glenoid with a finger, and this allows easier placement of retractors to expose the glenoid. This step when first tried seems a difficult manoeuvre and the difficulties we believe result in a number of proposed total shoulder replacements becoming hemiarthro-

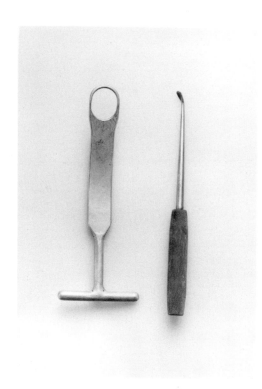

Figure 4.9 Fukuda ring retractor (left) and Fisher curette (right) – useful instruments for shoulder arthroplasty.

plasties through an inability to visualize the glenoid. The key to a good exposure lies in the position of the arm abduction and on good retraction. A ring retractor of the Fukuda type is invaluable (Figure 4.9). When this is placed on the posteroinferior lip of the glenoid and used to retract the humerus away, it allows excellent access to the whole glenoid. A Köbel-type retractor at the front of the glenoid completes the exposure. At this stage it is essential to separate the whole rotator cuff from the rim of the glenoid and the scapular neck to ensure full mobilization of the rotator cuff muscles. This is done by a combination of sharp and blunt dissection.

Preparation of the glenoid

Next, a template is used to cut the slot for the glenoid component and is orientated vertically using the posterior margin of the base of the coracoid process as the superior reference point. It is important to have an axial radiograph of the shoulder available in the operating room at this stage as osteophytes may shift the apparent centre of the glenoid anteriorly or

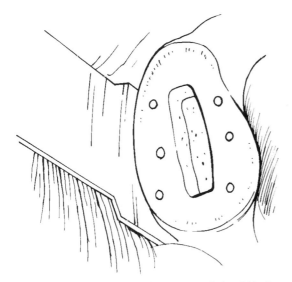

Figure 4.10 The appearance of the prepared glenoid before application of the cement and glenoid component.

joint becoming infected the resulting organisms have often been found to be antibiotic resistant (Lynch et al, 1987).

Preparation of the humerus

The preparation of the humerus is greatly facilitated by allowing the arm to hang vertically. The shaft is reamed using the sized reamers to allow insertion of the largest stem without breaching the humeral cortex. The reamers have a screw thread (Figure 4.11) and need to be rotated anticlockwise to remove them. The humeral head size chosen is the one which best fits the anatomy of the patient and allows the best tensioning of the rotator cuff. The large (22 mm) humeral head biomechanically improves the lever arm, thereby improving the efficiency of deltoid. The proximal part of the head should extend only slightly beyond the superior surface of the greater tuberosity so as not to stretch the superior cuff over its surface. The head of the prosthesis should be placed in 30–40° of retroversion. We now routinely cement **all** humeral components.

The lesser tuberosity is reattached using three

posteriorly, leading to an incorrect placement of the glenoid component. Preoperative radiographs will also indicate whether superior glenoid erosion has taken place and if this needs to be corrected. This is dealt with further in Chapter 7. The subchondral plate of the glenoid is broached using a high speed burr and the underlying cancellous bone excavated. Care should be taken with the burr as it is easy to break through the cortex of the glenoid neck. An angled Fisher curette (Figure 4.9) can now be used to complete the excavation into the base of the coracoid and down into the scapula. Any cartilage left on the remaining glenoid is removed with the burr and a number of small keyholes are placed in the subchondral bone to aid cement injection (Figure 4.10). The majority of the subchondral plate is left intact. Glenoid erosions may cause difficulties with seating of the implant and techniques have been described by Neer (1988) for dealing with these.

In most cases the metal-backed glenoid can be inserted, although we have had occasions to use the polyethylene component if the glenoid is very small, when the triangular peg of this component can be trimmed with scissors.

After thorough lavage of the bone and the optional use of hydrogen peroxide to reduce bleeding to a minimum the glenoid is inserted using bone cement. It is our practice not to use antibiotic-loaded cement in any primary arthroplasty, believing it offers no significant additional protection, and in the event of the

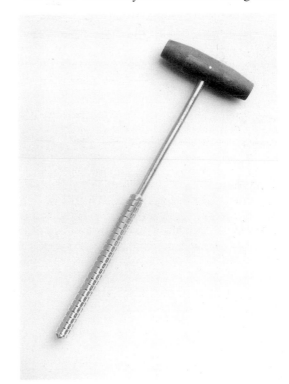

Figure 4.11 Humeral reamer with screw thread. This instrument should be used with care.

double-loop sutures of 1 PDS (polydioxanone). The suture is passed around the lesser tuberosity fragment and through the bony bed of the humerus so that it passes lateral to the cortical bicipital groove and is tied in front. The needle can be easily pushed through bone and no drill holes are needed. The rotator interval is closed with interrupted absorbable sutures and the deltoid and pectoralis major muscles are approximated over a suction drain. The skin is closed using a continuous subcuticular suture (either absorbable or 2/0 Proline suture removed at 10 days). The arm is placed in a broad arm-sling until removal of the drain at 48 hours.

Rehabilitation

In general we follow the guidelines laid down by Neer (Neer, Watson and Stanton, 1982) in the postoperative period. These are described in Chapter 6. We allow the patient to rest for 4 days before starting physiotherapy. Outpatient physiotherapy is commenced, paying particular attention to muscle strengthening exercises. Use is made of the hydrotherapy pool to provide resistance for the shoulder muscles. The patient is loaned a pulley to allow concentration on exercises at home. The quality of the result depends upon the dedication of the patient, and all patients are told that it will be at least a year before they will see the full benefit of the surgery.

Results

Neer (Neer, Watson and Stanton, 1982) published the results of 192 shoulder replacements reviewed after 24–99 months. Of 150 patients in the full exercise programme, that is those patients that had a good rotator cuff or a good repair of a rotator cuff, 86% achieved an excellent or satisfactory rating. A small group of patients were put into a limited goals rehabilitation category; and of these 44 patients 42 were described as successful, that is pain free with 20° of external rotation and 90° of elevation.

These results are excellent but results are dependent upon the selection of the patient, the skill of the surgeon, the physiotherapy facilities in any particular institution and the motivation of the patient. This is illustrated if one compares results published by Kelly, Foster and Fisher from Glasgow (1987), who reported on 42 shoulder replacements in 37 patients with rheumatoid arthritis. They felt that using Neer's classification only six patients would have achieved a satisfactory grading and that even using the limited goals criteria only 20 shoulders would have been graded successful. The principal reason they found for this poor result was the lack of elevation. By comparison, Neer (Neer, Watson and Stanton, 1982) reported 50 patients with total shoulder replacements for rheumatoid arthritis. Of these, 28 were graded excellent and 12 satisfactory, that is 80% of the patients fell into the satisfactory or excellent group. Neer only reported three unsatisfactory patients and it should be borne in mind that in his series 14 patients had full-thickness rotator cuff tears necessitating repair. Only eight of the patients in Kelly's series had full-thickness tears of the rotator cuff. Other authors have also failed to produce the impressive results that Neer has obtained. In 1986 we reported a series of 25 shoulders to the 3rd International Conference on Shoulder Surgery (Hirst and Wallace, 1986). Whilst overall the results were reasonable, the strikingly poor results were in those six shoulders with full-thickness rotator cuff tears. Several ways of repairing the tear where tried, including direct repair and fascia lata and Dacron grafts. These were universally unsuccessful and none of the patients would have been graded as satisfactory under even the limited goals criteria. Rotator cuff tears would seem to be the major limiting factor in the success of total shoulder replacements, and as yet no reliable way of dealing with these has been described. It remains to be seen whether or not synthetic replacements for the cuff, such as the Nottingham hood, will improve the objective results.

But perhaps we should not be too critical. All of the patients reported from Glasgow (Kelly, Foster and Fisher 1987) felt satisfied with the result despite the relatively poor objective findings. The poor scoring is probably due to the bias in Neer's scoring system on elevation despite the fact that very few daily activities are performed at or above shoulder height. Kelly's patient satisfaction was probably also a reflection of the success of the prosthesis in reducing pain (Sledge, 1980), something most patients with inflammatory joint disease are extremely grateful for.

Our recent results seem to be much better than those reported in 1986 and this would appear to stem from the remarkably few instances of rotator cuff tears in the rheumatoid population that we have dealt with and also to our being further up the learning curve. The learning curve for shoulder replacement would appear to be steep and the best results would seem to be obtained by surgeons with a greater experience of the technique and those working within centres with good facilities. We firmly believe that the postoperative rehabilitation period is critical to the success of a total shoulder replacement. The best results can only be achieved in centres where expertise is concentrated and particularly where the physiotherapy and rehabilitation staff are skilled in dealing with shoulder replacements. It should also be noted that the shoulder function continues to improve for a significant period of time and most of our patients do not peak until at least 1 year after surgery.

Loosening does not appear to be a major problem, indeed Neer (Neer, Watson and Stanton, 1982) has reported no instance of early clinical loosening and this has been confirmed by Kelly (Kelly, Foster and Fisher, 1987). Despite significant numbers of radiolucent lines around the glenoid component Neer (1988) has reported no reoperation for loosening of the components in a series of 661 humeral and 517 glenoid components with an average follow-up of 6 years. It would seem that, in terms of loosening, the prosthesis is durable. However, no evidence is yet available on the effects of wear of the components.

Whatever the quality of the results from individual units, we would echo the plea from Johnston et al (1990) that a uniformity of reporting is necessary to enable comparisons to be made between differing prostheses and operative techniques. Without this, no meaningful conclusions can be drawn from the various published data, and no sensible progress will be made. It is yet to be seen whether the new shoulder evaluation method of Constant (Chapter 3) will replace that of Cofield's rating sheets (Neer, Watson and Stanton, 1982), which had become the standard assessment forms in the 1980s. The Constant evaluation sheets have now received the full support of the European Society for the Study of the Shoulder and Elbow.

References

Hirst P and Wallace WA (1986) Poor results of Neer shoulder replacement in rheumatoid arthritis. *Proceedings of the 3rd International Conference on Surgery of the Shoulder*, pp. 362–366.

Johnston RC, Fitzgerald RH, Harris WH, Poss R, Müller ME and Sledge CB (1990) Clinical and radiographic evaluation of total hip replacement. *Journal of Bone and Joint Surgery* **72A** 161–168.

Kelly IG, Foster RS and Fisher WD (1987) Neer total shoulder replacement in rheumatoid arthritis. *Journal of Bone and Joint Surgery* **69B** 723–726.

Lettin AWF, Copeland SA and Scales JT (1982) The Stanmore total shoulder replacement. *Journal of Bone and Joint Surgery* **64B** 47–51.

Lidwell OM, Lowbury EJL, Whyte W, Blowers R, Stanley SJ and Lowe D (1983) Ventilation in operating rooms *BMJ* **286** 1214–1215.

Lynch M, Esser MP, Shelley P and Wroblewski BM (1987) Deep infection in Charnley low friction arthroplasty. *Journal of Bone and Joint Surgery* **69B** 355–360.

Neer CS (1988) Non-constrained shoulder arthroplasty: indications and special steps in technique. In *Current Trends in Orthopaedic Surgery* (CSB Galasko and J Noble, eds), pp. 12–24. Manchester: Manchester University Press.

Neer CS, Watson KC and Stanton FJ (1982) Recent experiences in total shoulder replacement. *Journal of Bone and Joint Surgery* **64A** 319–337.

Neviaser RJ and Neviaser TJ (1985) Major ruptures of the rotator cuff. In *Practical Shoulder Surgery* (M Watson, ed.), pp. 171–224. London: Grune and Stratton.

Sledge CB (1980) Shoulder replacement arthroplasty. *Orthopäde* **9** 177–184.

5

Total shoulder replacement in rheumatoid arthritis

Ian G. Kelly

Shoulder pain has been estimated to occur in between 58 and 89% (Petersson, 1986; Gschwend, 1988) of all rheumatoid patients. Not all of these patients will require 'shoulder' arthroplasty, either because their symptoms can be adequately managed by non-operative means or because they are experiencing pain from the extra glenohumeral articulations of the shoulder joint complex – the acromioclavicular and subacromial joints. However, the frequency with which the glenohumeral joint is involved in rheumatoid arthritis results in this disease providing the major indication for shoulder arthroplasty in Great Britain and Europe.

Classification of glenohumeral disease

The pathology of the rheumatoid shoulder is highly variable and in order to permit comparison between different series of patients some form of classification must be used. The surgeon requires to know:

- The pathological anatomy of the shoulder.
- The rate of progression of the disease process.
- The functional state of the patient.
- The functional state of the shoulder.

Although several radiological and functional classifications are in existence very few authors have made use of them. I will outline the approach to classification that I employ but would emphasize the need for a universally accepted system.

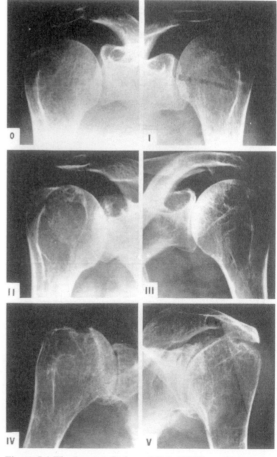

Figure 5.1 The Larsen, Dale and Eek (1977) grading system for the rheumatoid glenohumeral joint. Note the large erosions and joint space narrowing in grade III, the severe destructive changes in grade IV and the gross disorganization of the joint in grade V.

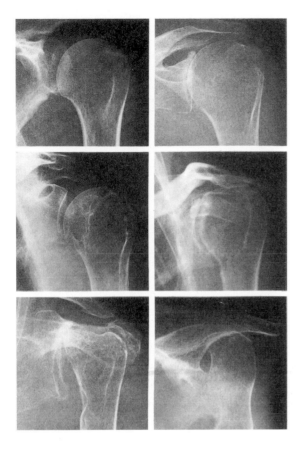

Figure 5.2 Jónsson's modification of the Larsen system (Jónsson, 1988). Stage 1 includes minor erosions and obliteration of the joint space. Stage 2 has severe osteoporosis, cysts and erosions with attrition of the humeral head and glenoid. Stage 3 is the end-stage shoulder with marked destruction. (Reproduced with permission from Jónsson, 1988.)

For technical reasons it is important to assess the degree of destruction that has taken place at the glenohumeral joint. Of the several available radiological classifications (Crossan and Vallance, 1982; Dijkstra et al, 1985) that of Larsen, Dale and Eek (1977) is the most widely quoted (Figure 5.1). It is part of their wider system of joint staging in rheumatoid arthritis. There are five grades which reflect the progression of the destruction at the glenohumeral joint. This system of grading is widely used by rheumatologists and provides a means by which clinical material may be compared. However, as far as surgical intervention, and arthroplasty in particular, is concerned most shoulders are in grades III–V. Jónsson (1988) has modified the Larsen system for surgical use and has proposed a three-stage system, as follows (Figure 5.2):

- *Stage 1* Narrowed joint space; the subchondral bone of the humeral head is intact but there may be slight erosions at the anatomical neck and superior subluxation.
- *Stage 2* The humeral head is reasonably spherical despite attrition, cysts and erosions.
- *Stage 3* The humeral head is severely destroyed with neoarticulation at the humeral neck.

This closely mirrors my personal experience of the rheumatoid glenohumeral joint from a surgical viewpoint but until Jónsson's system is more widely recognized it is probably better to employ the more commonly used Larsen classification.

The rate of progression of the disease process is important both from the point of view of planning treatment and with regard to the state of the soft tissues. Although the level of general disease activity, as indicated by the sedimentation rate or the C-reactive protein levels, may reflect the disease in the shoulder, this is not always the case. I have found Neer's approach to the grading of the rheumatoid shoulder to be of considerable value. Neer (1990) describes three types of rheumatoid shoulder – dry, wet and resorptive – each of which may be low-grade, intermediate or severe.

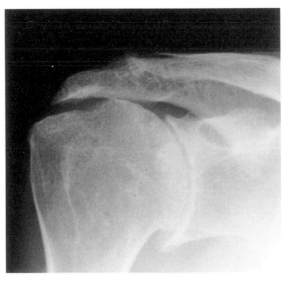

Figure 5.3 The 'dry' form of Neer's system (1990) of classifying the rheumatoid glenohumeral joint. Note the secondary osteoarthritic features.

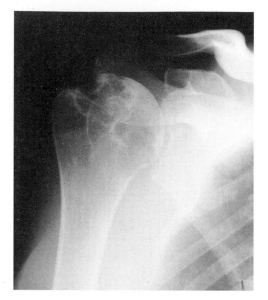

Figure 5.4 The 'wet' form of rheumatoid shoulder according to Neer (1990). The active synovitis has resulted in large erosions of the humeral head.

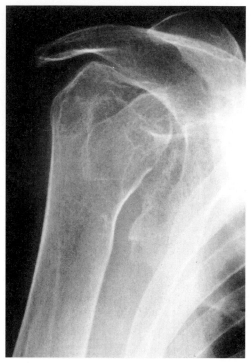

Figure 5.5 The 'resorptive' type of glenohumeral disease (Neer 1982) showing the end-stage shoulder.

The dry form (Figure 5.3) has sclerosis, subchondral cysts and loss of joint space. Erosions are minimal and osteophytes are common. The joint is stiff. Progress is not rapid and may arrest without major bone loss. The rotator cuff is usually intact.

The wet shoulder (Figure 5.4) has exuberant synovium causing erosions and severe bone destruction. This type of shoulder may show rapid progress of bony destruction with early rupture of the rotator cuff.

In the resorptive form (Figure 5.5) there is extensive bone loss but little bony reaction. The rotator cuff usually remains intact but may be severely attenuated.

The end-stage shoulder can result from either the resorptive or the wet forms of the disease. It is characterized by articulation of the inferior pole of the glenoid (almost always preserved in rheumatoid arthritis) and the shaft of the humerus. The rotator cuff is usually, but not always, ruptured.

This classification is based upon clinical experience and there are few studies of the natural history of the rheumatoid shoulder. Petersson (1986), in a study of 105 rheumatoid patients, showed a correlation between the duration of the disease and the extent of the radiological changes and concluded that there was an inexorable downhill course towards joint destruction and incapacity in many

patients. Crossan and Vallance (1982) followed 20 painful shoulders with little joint damage by means of a retrospective radiological review. Five shoulders showed an increase in the size of the erosions but the remaining 15 progressed to severe or end-stage damage with either acute (3) or chronic (12) superior subluxation of the humeral head. Two of the three shoulders with acute subluxation underwent arthrography and both showed the presence of a rotator cuff tear, which was confirmed to be massive in one at later exploration. The chronic group showed progression over a period of 2–3 years and the subluxation was associated with distortion of the humeral head. Both of these reports considered all rheumatoid shoulders to be the same and therefore fail to provide the surgeon with a method of identifying those shoulders which will progress rapidly.

Using the Neer types in our own unit, we have found that the rates of progression differ according to the type. In a group of 56 shoulders followed for between two and six years radiological progression was seen in 6 of 7 wet shoulders, none of 16 with the dry pattern and 9 of 30 shoulders with the resorptive pattern.

In a study of 104 patients undergoing shoulder arthroplasty, cuff rupture was found in 21 of 30 wet shoulders, 2 of 10 dry shoulders, 4 of 56 resorptive shoulders and 4 of 8 end stage shoulders. Forty three of the resorptive shoulders had thin rotator cuffs. Further, all but 15 shoulders were reported as having deficient glenoid bone. All 15 were in the wet group. Thus, shoulders with the wet pattern progress more rapidly, have a higher risk of rupturing the rotator cuff and may rupture the cuff before there is significant loss of glenoid bone.

The functional status of the entire patient must be considered as this may dictate the function required at the shoulder. At present the most widely quoted functional grading system is that of the American Rheumatology Association (ARA) (Steinbrocker, Traeger and Batterman, 1949):

- *Grade I* Capable of all activities.
- *Grade II* Moderate restrictions – adequate for normal activities.
- *Grade III* Marked restrictions – self-care only.
- *Grade IV* Bed and/or chair – little or no self-care.

Although this is a useful method of grouping rheumatoid patients whose disabilities frequently result from involvement of more than one joint, it is a crude system as applied to the functions of any particular joint. My personal preference is for the capability to perform individual activities of daily living to be recorded so that the effect of any therapeutic

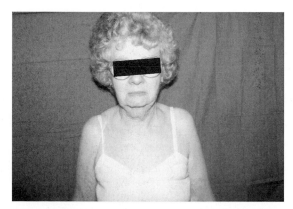

Figure 5.6 Medialization of the glenohumeral joint. Note the apparent deltoid wasting on the left.

measure may be seen but to consider these together with the ARA grade. I do not believe that the use of assessment systems which present the results of clinical, radiological and functional status as a single figure score may not be as useful for a comparison of different series.

Indications for surgery

The indications for shoulder arthroplasty are usually given as being severe pain and marked impairment of function in a patient with arthritis of the shoulder. In rheumatoid arthritis this is an oversimplification. Rheumatoid arthritis is a polyarthritis and as such it can affect any or all of the components of the shoulder joint complex. Severe pain and limited function can result from involvement of the acromioclavicular joint and/or subacromial region as well as from disease of the glenohumeral joint.

Glenohumeral arthroplasty can only be considered a logical treatment if the glenohumeral joint is the source of the pain and limited movements. The site of the pain in the rheumatoid shoulder is a poor guide to the joints that are involved (Kelly, 1990a): most rheumatoid patients complain of pain over the point of the shoulder and anteriorly which radiates towards the deltoid insertion irrespective of the radiological pattern of joint disease. Radiographs, whilst they show the distribution and extent of the bony changes, give no indication of the site of pain. On clinical examination, medialization of the shoulder resulting from destruction of the glenoid and/or humeral head (Figure 5.6) and lack of external rotation are the most useful signs of significant disease in the glenohumeral joint. In my experience the most useful way of identifying the site of the pain is the use of local anaesthetic injections.

Testing is performed by the injection of no more than 1 ml 1% lignocaine into the subacromial region, the acromioclavicular joint or the glenohumeral joint. In a typical test either the subacromial region or the acromioclavicular joint would be injected first. It is necessary to wait for at least 3 minutes to allow the local anaesthetic to act. The patient is then asked to put the limb through a range of movement and any change in the level of the pain or the range of movement is noted. If there has been complete relief of pain the test is concluded, otherwise it proceeds with injection of the next extra-glenohumeral joint. The test is completed when pain relief is achieved or when the glenohumeral joint has been injected.

Correlation of the patient's description of the pain, the physical signs, the radiographic appearances and the results of the injection studies in 75 rheumatoid patients with painful shoulders indicates that, when the glenohumeral joint is implicated as the site of pain, humeral head sphericity has usually been lost on the radiographs and external rotation remains limited despite injection. Thus, my indications for glenohumeral arthroplasty in rheumatoid arthritis are injection studies implicating the glenohumeral joint accompanied by loss of sphericity of the humeral head on the radiographs (Larsen grade V). If the glenohumeral joint is implicated but the humeral head sphericity and external rotation are preserved – an unusual situation – synovectomy is probably indicated.

In addition to providing the indication for arthroplasty the injection studies also indicate which other components of the shoulder complex are contributing to the pain. These sites can then receive treatment at the same time as the glenohumeral joint, permitting the best possible result to be obtained from the surgery (see below).

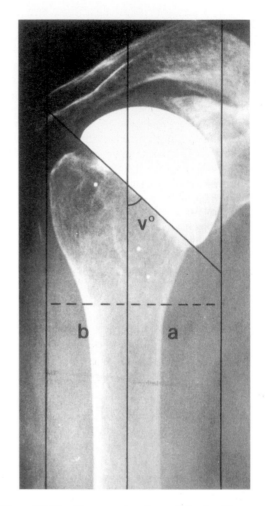

Figure 5.7 Metallic cup arthroplasty of the shoulder. (Reproduced with permission from Jónsson, 1988.)

Types of prostheses

Shoulder prostheses are usually divided into constrained, semiconstrained and unconstrained types.

The constrained forms include the Michael Reese (Post, Haskell and Jablon, 1980) and the Gristina trispherical prosthesis (Gristina and Webb, 1982). The so-called semiconstrained arthroplasties are typified by the Stanmore (Lettin, Copeland and Scales, 1982) and Kessel (Kessel and Bayley, 1979) prostheses. These last devices, although they are not as constrained as those in the first group, have been designed with a considerable amount of constraint and I prefer to consider them along with the constrained prostheses.

Initially these prostheses comprised a stemmed humeral component articulating with a cup which was fixed to the glenoid using a stem or pegs. However, problems with glenoid fixation resulted in new designs which reversed the ball and socket, with the latter being placed in the humerus, e.g. the Kessel prosthesis. Problems with fractures led to modifications in design to allow prosthetic failure, that is dislocation, to take place rather than bony failure. Reported experience of this group of prostheses in rheumatoid arthritis is limited.

Better appreciation of the factors contributing to the stability of the glenohumeral joint and the realization that the majority of shoulders have an intact rotator cuff resulted in the development of unconstrained prostheses, of which the Neer device (Neer et al 1982) is the best known. This comprises a cobalt chrome-stemmed humeral head replace-

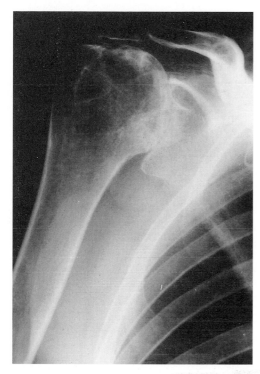

Figure 5.8 Larsen grade IV glenohumeral joint with superior subluxation and erosion of the superior portion of the glenoid. Note the sparing of the inferior pole of the glenoid.

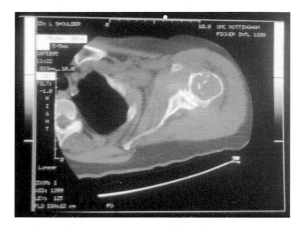

Figure 5.9 Computerized tomogram of the rheumatoid glenohumeral joint, showing the destruction of the glenoid, osteophyte formation and erosions and cyst formation on the humeral head.

ment and a polyethylene glenoid spacer. The majority of the reports in the literature concerning arthroplasty of the rheumatoid shoulder involve this type of prosthesis.

In recent years there has been a move towards modular forms of the unconstrained prosthesis. This has advantages with regard to the amount of bone stock to be retained but also facilitates soft tissue tensioning and revision surgery if necessary.

Resurfacing of the humeral head using a cup also provides an unconstrained arthroplasty. The initial reports concerned the use of a silicone rubber cup (Varian, 1980) used in 32 arthroplasties in 29 patients, with good pain relief but little improvement in the range of glenohumeral movement. This prosthesis has proved difficult to fix in place and the silicone rubber has not proved suitable for use in this site. Steffee and Moore (1984) reported the use of an Indiana hip cup at the shoulder and introduced a purpose-built shoulder cup. Jónsson et al (1986) reported the use of a similar metallic cup, fixed to the humerus with bone cement, in 26 shoulders in 24 rheumatoid patients (Figure 5.7).

Operative pathology of the rheumatoid shoulder

Unconstrained arthroplasties depend upon the presence of a functioning rotator cuff and deltoid muscle for satisfactory function. Rheumatoid disease involves all tissues and poor muscle and an abnormal cuff are commonly present. The appearances of superior subluxation of the humeral head on radiographs of the rheumatoid shoulder resulted in the belief that rotator cuff rupture was commonly present. However, studies by Neer et al (1982), Cofield (1984), Kelly, Foster and Fisher (1987), Barrett et al (1987) and Sledge et al (1989) have demonstrated that between 70 and 80% of rheumatoid shoulders have intact rotator cuffs, although in only about 20% are these cuffs normal. The most common abnormality is thinning of the cuff and the superior subluxation seen on the radiographs is probably due to a combination of this and the cephalic erosion of the glenoid (see below).

The state of the deltoid muscle is not often quoted but I have been surprised how often it is of good quality. In a series of 71 rheumatoid shoulders undergoing arthroplasty (all Larsen grades IV or V), 41 were reported to have normal deltoid muscles (Kelly, 1990b). This may be particularly notable in those patients with severe medialization of their shoulders, emphasizing that the deformity is mainly due to bone loss and not muscle wasting.

Loss of bone stock is an inevitable accompaniment of rheumatoid involvement of the glenohumeral joint, although this may be of mild degree. Medialization of the glenoid without excessive anterior or posterior erosion is commonly seen, especially in the dry type of disease, and in this situation the humeral head is usually preserved. More major humeral head or glenoid bone loss may be seen with active synovitis. In both types of disease glenoid destruction results in a cephalad orientation of the glenoid face, with the superior portion of the glenoid being eroded towards the base of the coracoid, whilst the inferior margin is often unaffected (Figure 5.8). Beddow (1988), using computerized tomography, has reported that the pattern of glenoid destruction varies between osteoarthritis and rheumatoid arthritis only in degree (Figure 5.9). A similar study of the humeral head by Jónsson (1988) has revealed the frequent occurrence of cysts, some of which may be very large and communicate with the joint cavity. Since most arthroplasties involve the resection of the humeral head, this only becomes of significance if a cup resurfacing procedure is to be used.

The tendon of the long head of biceps, a depressor of the humeral head, may be damaged as part of the rheumatoid process but, like the deltoid muscle, its status is rarely recorded. In my own series, 14 of 71 were noted to be intact.

The degree and activity of the synovitis is extremely variable, but is more likely to be marked in the wet pattern. Capsular laxity varies with the degree of synovitis and the capsule is usually adherent to the tendon of subscapularis so that the two are divided as one layer when entering the glenohumeral joint. The coracoacromial ligament is usually intact unless there has been a long-standing major rotator cuff tear or previous surgery, and a large thickened subacromial bursa is encountered only infrequently.

Surgical technique

Total shoulder arthroplasty in this group of patients is performed much in the same way as in any other condition. However, the pathological changes that may be present can cause difficulties and the surgery can be made easier by the use of several modifications to the operative technique.

I prefer to use the beach chair position for this procedure, using a neurosurgical headrest to support the head. Preoperative flexion and extension lateral radiographs of the cervical spine are essential so that the anaesthetist knows the degree of neck flexion that is safe and the surgeon can place the head in a suitable position. This systemic disease produces thinning of the skin and most of the patients are thin so attention must be paid to adequate padding over bony points, such as the elbows and heels, to prevent pressure sores developing. A small surgical drape folded and placed medial to the medial border of the scapula will facilitate later access to the glenoid.

I employ an anterior approach to the shoulder, as described by Neer (1982), dividing only the tendon of the subscapularis. The medialization of so many of the glenohumeral joints makes access difficult unless the deltoid is carefully elevated from the underlying humerus by blunt dissection using the index finger. The muscle is not detached from the acromion or the humerus and care must be taken to ensure that all of the fibres of deltoid are elevated *en masse* to avoid damage to the axillary nerve. The finger is passed posterior to the shaft of the humerus as far distal as the deltoid insertion and proximally into the subacromial space. An Aufranc bone lever can then be inserted into the subacromial region, giving good exposure with a small degree of abduction and serving to protect the muscle. Detachment of the coracoid process and its muscles is virtually never necessary.

The coracoacromial ligament serves to prevent superior subluxation of the humeral head – an appearance which may be associated with deficiency of the rotator cuff – and I prefer to leave it intact if at all possible. If the cuff is torn, section of the ligament will be necessary to facilitate the repair.

The majority of rheumatoid patients undergoing shoulder arthroplasty have severe restriction of external rotation or even fixed internal rotation deformities. It is therefore necessary to gain length in subscapularis if external rotation is to be restored postoperatively. Neer (1990) has described a Z-plasty of the subscapularis tendon which is useful in patients with osteoarthritis or post-traumatic problems but inappropriate in most rheumatoid shoulders, where the tendon is thin. Fortunately, adequate lengthening can usually be achieved by freeing

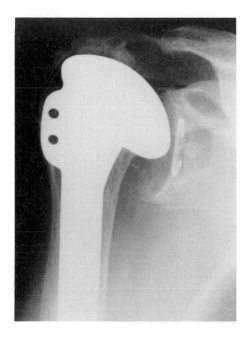

Fig. 5.10 Superior subluxation of the humeral head with sclerosis on the underside of the acromion. The rotator cuff was not functional. Note that the outer end of the clavicle has been resected and that the tip of the glenoid component has been removed to accommodate it within the bony glenoid.

cing it. I do not think that building up the defect with bone cement is an acceptable form of management because early failure of the unconstrained cement is likely. If glenoid bone stock is so poor that a prosthesis cannot be inserted, a satisfactory result can be obtained from humeral head replacement alone but the surgeon must ensure that the surface of the glenoid bone is smooth and as congruous as possible with the prosthetic humeral head.

The polyarthritic nature of rheumatoid disease must not be forgotten and the management of the acromioclavicular and subacromial articulations must be considered if the best possible result is to be achieved. I have already indicated that local anaesthetic injection studies provide the basis for my decision regarding the treatment of these joints. Excision of the outer end of the clavicle is frequently indicated but I do not favour anterior acromioplasty unless the underside of the acromion is markedly irregular. Insertion of the humeral prosthesis proud of the greater tuberosity should prevent any postoperative subacromial impingement. If acromioplasty is performed an attempt should be made to reattach the coracoacromial ligament, although this can be very difficult if the bone is soft and thin.

Results of shoulder arthroplasty

The results of the various types of arthroplasty are usually presented for pain, range of movement and function. However, all of these factors must be considered according to the diagnosis, the class of prosthesis (constrained, unconstrained or surface), whether or not the glenoid is resurfaced (total or hemiarthroplasty) and the pathological status of the shoulder – most importantly whether the rotator cuff is diseased. Comparison between series and prostheses is made difficult or impossible by the differing methods of presenting results or the failure to provide details of the patient group.

Constrained prostheses

This group includes the Kessel (Kessel and Bayley, 1979), Stanmore (Coughlin, Morris and West, 1979; Lettin, Copeland and Scales, 1982)

the combined subscapularis and capsule from the anterior glenoid after section of the humeral head. In order to achieve adequate external rotation it may be necessary to use a thinner prosthetic humeral head, although it is clearly essential to tension the cuff adequately.

I prefer to prepare the glenoid after resection of the humeral head but before reaming the humerus. If the humerus is reamed first there is a danger of crushing the thin humeral bone while it is being retracted. Severe erosion of the glenoid bone is commonly encountered in these patients. The typical glenoid has medialized towards the coracoid and has a mild cephalic tilt (see Figure 5.8). If the fin of the Neer non-metal-backed glenoid component cannot be accommodated by the glenoid bone, the tip may be cut off (Figure 5.10). Fortunately, severe anterior or posterior erosion is uncommon, but if encountered it necessitates the attachment of a piece of iliac crest bone using AO screws to provide a platform for the prosthesis or the judicious use of a burr to realign the face of the glenoid before resurfa-

and the Michael Reese (Post, Haskell and Jablon, 1980; Post and Jablon, 1983) devices. The last is a linked prosthesis which allows dislocation to occur once a certain torque value is exceeded, whereas the first two designs incorporate a ball and socket. In the case of the Kessel prosthesis the ball is mounted on the scapula.

Eight shoulders with rheumatoid arthritis are included in the material managed with the Michael Reese prosthesis (Post and Jablon, 1983) but the results were not analysed separately. This series comprised patients treated with the original prosthesis (series I) and those who received the modified version with improved glenoid fixation (series II). All but two of the shoulders were said to have 'poor to absent function of the short rotators'. Pain relief for the entire group was good in the majority but a large number of shoulders required revision. Function and ranges of movement were considered to be the same, and for the series II patients (seven of the rheumatoid shoulders were in this group) there was '60% overall improvement in active function and a 65% gain in passive function'. Although there is a relationship between range of movement and function they are clearly not the same (Badley, Wagstaff and Wood, 1984) and function in rheumatoid patients will also depend upon the state of other joints. Of the 24 series I shoulders, 11 were revised: three for infection and the others for bending or breaking of the prosthetic humeral neck. Eight of the 78 shoulders with series II prostheses required revision, seven of which were for dislocation. At radiological examination 2 years after operation 50% showed radiolucency about the humeral stem and 30% radiolucency about the glenoid screws and central post. The authors indicated that the glenoid bone must not be severely eroded or porotic if this prosthesis is to be used and they recommended that unconstrained arthroplasty be used if the rotator cuff is, or can be made, functional.

In a preliminary communication on his prosthesis Kessel (Kessel and Bayley, 1979) reported the early results of surgery in 24 shoulders performed over a 5-year period, 17 of which were in rheumatoid patients. Four were excluded because of inadequate duration of review, and two died. The results for the entire group indicated that pain relief was satisfactory in all but two shoulders. Function improved in 11 shoulders and active motion was increased in 12 shoulders. Two shoulders underwent revision: one for glenoid loosening and the other for malalignment and dislocation. There were also two instances of late dislocation.

The Stanmore prosthesis was used in five rheumatoid shoulders in Coughlin's 17 cases (Coughlin, Morris and West, 1979) and 34 rheumatoid shoulders in Lettin's 50 arthroplasties (Lettin, Copeland and Scales 1982). Coughlin reported the results according to the aetiology of the arthritis and found that the greatest *increase* in 'total range of motion' was seen in the patients with rheumatoid arthritis, although the postoperative total range was almost the same for the rheumatoid and osteoarthritic groups. Most patients were said to show an increase in their daily activity postoperatively. Pain relief was complete in 50% of patients, and patient satisfaction, calculated on the basis of pain relief, function of the involved limb and decreased reliance on analgesics, was greatest in the rheumatoid patient.

In Lettin's series all but nine of the patients had satisfactory pain relief. Abduction, flexion and external rotation averaged gains of 20°, while internal rotation improved by an average of 40°. An 'elaborate series' of functional tests was used but little change was seen in the activities before and after the operation. There was, however, a marked increase in the number of patients who could perform specific tasks after surgery.

Coughlin noted only one case of loosening, whereas Lettin found loosening of the glenoid component in ten patients, in eight of whom the cup was replaced. Six of these patients later developed loosening of the revised cup. Lettin also reported dislocation in three patients and deep infection in one. Nine patients were left with an excision arthroplasty and their range of movement was no worse than that before the initial surgery. Six of these patients were virtually pain free.

Constraint, while compensating for absent rotator cuff function, places increased stresses on the glenoid and this results in failure, especially if the bone is deficient or porotic. The place of these prostheses is therefore extremely limited in rheumatoid arthritis, even when the rotator cuff is irreparable.

Table 5.1 Humeral head replacement in rheumatoid arthritis: ranges of movement (degrees)

Author(s)	n	Flexion	Abduction	Ext. rot.	Int. rot.	Extension
Marmor (1977)	12	—	80(32)	—	—	—
Varian (1980)						
Clayton, Ferlic and Jeffers (1982)	7	—(19)	—	—(15)	—(19)	—
Bodey and Yeoman (1983)	6	—	66(13)	—	60(20)	—
Jónsson et al (1986)	26	66(36)	57(33)	59(50)	32(27)	44(34)

Values in parentheses represent gain in motion.
Ext. rot., external rotation; Int. rot., internal rotation.

Table 5.2 Unconstrained total shoulder arthroplasty in rheumatoid arthritis (Neer design): ranges of movement (degrees)

Author(s)	n	Flexion	Abduction	Ext. rot.	Int. rot.	Extension
Neer et al (1982)	43	—(57)	—	—(60)	—	—
Cofield (1984)	29	—	103(46)	35(—)	*	—
Pahle and Kvarnes (1985)	41	—(16)	—(24)	—(15)	—(6)	—(13)
Kelly, Foster and Fisher (1987)	42	75(20)	—	40(29)	*	50(32)
Barrett et al (1987)	11	100(34)	—	—(16)	*	—
Sledge et al (1989)	122	90(34)	—	40(20)	—	—
Hawkins, Bell and Jallay (1989)	34	100(42)	—	35(13)	—	—
Kelly (1990b)	71	79(15)	—	39(29)	*	55(15)

Values in parentheses represent gains in motion.
Ext. rot., external rotation; Int. rot., internal rotation.
*Internal rotation expressed as the anatomical segment reached with the hand.

Table 5.3 Function after shoulder arthroplasty (all designs)

Author(s)	n	Perineal care	Opposite axilla	Comb hair	Hand at shoulder level	Hand above shoulder level
Jónsson et al (1986)	26	26	—	—	—	—
Kelly, Foster and Fisher (1987)	42	34	39	22	29	12
Barrett et al (1987)	11	11	11	8	8	—
Sledge et al (1989)	122	102	—	80	84	—
Roper, Paterson and Day (1990)	25*	18	18	4	—	—
Kelly (1990b)	71	54	—	44	44	—

*Functional results quoted for all 25 patients, 18 of whom suffered rheumatoid arthritis.

Unconstrained prostheses

Humeral head replacement

Neer's initial prosthesis (Neer, 1955) merely replaced the humeral head, but this series of 12 patients did not include any with rheumatoid arthritis. The results for the use of 'hemiarthroplasty' in rheumatoid patients are shown in Table 5.1. The majority of these reports refer to the use of the Neer humeral component but note should be made of the cup arthroplasty reported by Jónsson et al (1986) and the Silastic cup used by Varian (1980). The results of Jónsson's prosthesis are similar to those of the stemmed prostheses but the presence of large cysts in the humeral head may militate against its use in some patients.

Since rheumatoid arthritis affects both surfaces of the glenohumeral joint, merely replacing the humeral head appears to be illogical. However, my own experience suggests that this is an acceptable form of management as long as there is reasonable congruity between the glenoid and the prosthetic humeral head.

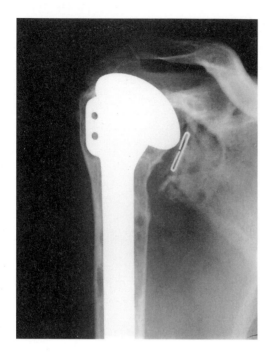

Figure 5.11. Cephalic orientation of the glenoid component with 'translocation' of the humeral head. Note the radiolucency at the glenoid cement–bone interface and the endosteal erosions within the humerus. Repeated aspiration and biopsy of the erosions has failed to establish the presence of infection. The patient is currently asymptomatic.

Total shoulder replacement

In his report on the use of humeral head replacement for the treatment of glenohumeral osteoarthritis, Neer (1974) mentioned the use of a polyethylene glenoid spacer anchored to the glenoid bone with bone cement. He was circumspect about the place of this component in osteoarthritis. However, resurfacing of the glenoid is now the norm in glenohumeral arthroplasty. Studies by Gschwend and Bischof (1991) suggest that, although the objective results do not differ between total and hemiarthroplasty, a large majority of patients prefer the total shoulder replacement.

The results for unconstrained glenohumeral arthroplasty in rheumatoid arthritis (Table 5.2) are generally inferior to those for osteoarthritis in terms of range of movement; this is almost certainly due to the high incidence of bone and rotator cuff deficiency in these patients. The movements obtained and the pain relief achieved permit the majority of these patients to experience a great functional improvement.

Because of the different methods used to quantify this, it is difficult to express the cumulative functional results in a standard form (Table 5.3). Further, since the state of the other upper limb joints and the joints of the lower limb affect the patient's function, it is difficult to compare patients.

The 'typical' rheumatoid patient will achieve 90° flexion, 40° external rotation, internal rotation sufficient to permit perineal care, almost total pain relief and major functional improvements.

Radiological assessment

The significance of the radiological appearance of cemented arthroplasties has been established by studies at the hip and knee (Tibrewal, Grant and Goodfellow, 1984), and the same principles have been applied to the shoulder. Radiographs are inspected for the alignment of the prostheses, radiolucent cement–prosthesis–bone lines and evidence of component migration.

Alignment of the prosthetic components will be influenced by their operative placement and, especially in rheumatoid arthritis, by the state of the rotator cuff.

The humeral component may be placed in inadequate or excessive retroversion, which may predispose to dislocation, or it may be inserted such that it lies distal to the greater tuberosity, resulting in subacromial impingement. The glenoid component may be seated high or low in the glenoid bone but more commonly in rheumatoid arthritis it lies in the plane of the eroded glenoid and is angled in a cephalic direction. This leads to superior translocation of the humeral head on the glenoid (Figure 5.11), a situation which will predispose to impingement and reduce the range of elevation.

Superior subluxation of the glenohumeral joint is commonly seen in rheumatoid arthritis (Kelly, Foster and Fisher, 1987) (Figure 5.10) and, as in the preoperative radiographs, it does not always indicate cuff rupture. It appears to be associated with the attenuated nature of the rotator cuff and I have found that the degree of subluxation can be reduced by preserving the coracoacromial ligament (Kelly, Foster and Fisher, 1987).

The presence of radiolucent lines at the cement–bone junction around the glenoid component has received considerable attention. Neer (1982) reports a 30% incidence but Cofield (1984), Amstutz, Sew Hoy and Clarke (1981), Kelly, Foster and Fisher (1987), Barrett et al (1987) and Sledge et al (1989) all report lucencies in approximately 80% of their shoulders in patients with rheumatoid arthritis – a figure not dissimilar to that seen in patients with osteoarthritis. Barrett's group found a relationship between the presence of a deficient rotator cuff and the incidence of glenoid lucencies, hypothesizing that the deficient cuff results in a more cephalic inclination of the resultant glenohumeral joint force, which then acts eccentrically on the glenoid component, producing a turning moment. They also felt that it was important to differentiate between lucencies around the flange of the Neer II prosthesis and those around the keel because only the latter were associated with loosening of the glenoid component in their series. Kelly (1990a), in a study of 71 Neer total shoulder replacement in rheumatoid patients followed for an average of 5.5 years, found that no glenoid lucent line showed progression beyond 2 years.

Migration of either of the components is an unusual event and can be very difficult to identify at an early stage. Jónsson (1989) has used stereophotogrammetry with tantalum balls implanted into the humerus and glenoid bone at the time of surgery to study the movements of his cup arthroplasty. His results indicate the quality of humeral head cup fixation but the technique, while requiring complex and expensive equipment, could be used to study total shoulder replacement.

Complications

The complications of unconstrained shoulder arthroplasty in rheumatoid arthritis encompass all of those encountered in other diagnostic groups, including infection, intraoperative fracture, instability and loosening. Despite the higher incidence of prosthetic infection seen in this group of patients after hip and knee surgery (Poss et al, 1984), no such trend is evident at the shoulder. In part this may be because the rarity of infection about shoulder arthroplasties makes it necessary for many cases to be studied before significant differences can be identified. However, the osteoporosis

which is usually present does appear to predispose towards intraoperative fractures and both the surgeon and assistant must be aware of this danger.

In my experience the most common complication encountered after shoulder arthroplasty in the rheumatoid patient is failure of the rotator cuff. This may occur as an acute episode but more usually presents as inability of the patient to perform actively the range of motion achieved passively during the initial period of rehabilitation and this may not become apparent for 6 or more weeks after surgery. A few of these patients have had rotator cuff tears repaired but the majority have merely been recorded as having an attenuated or thin cuff at operation. The previously intact but thin cuff may either rupture or be incapable of functioning adequately and for this reason I prefer to refer to this problem as 'non-function of the rotator cuff'. Although it may be worthwhile attempting repair when there has been an acute episode, my only experience of this was unsuccessful. The more insidious presentation causes the patient to have much reduced movements against gravity but has little effect upon function below shoulder level. For this reason and since the quality of the tendon is invariably poor, I do not advocate surgical intervention in these patients.

Survivorship analysis has been applied to shoulder arthroplasty (Brenner et al, 1989) and in a group of 51 shoulder arthroplasties followed for a minimum of 2 years (average 67 months) survivorship at 11 years was 73% for all prostheses and diagnostic groups and 92% for all prostheses in rheumatoid patients (25 shoulders). The authors do not discuss the reasons for the better survival figures in rheumatoid arthritis but they are likely to be related to the lower levels of physical demand made on their shoulders by these patients and the protective effect of disease at other upper limb joints.

Conclusion

Glenohumeral arthroplasty in the rheumatoid patient is now well established, well documented and has a high rate of success. Like other arthroplasties it results in excellent pain relief, but the state of the rotator cuff, its muscles and the deltoid muscle often dictate that little more than 90° of flexion can be achieved. Nevertheless, the improvement in rotations is great and this contributes towards the marked functional improvement that is seen. Complications are few and durability is notable. Shoulder arthroplasty is at least as successful as hip arthroplasty and is a very valuable part of any rheumatoid surgeon's armamentarium.

References

Amstutz HC, Sew Hoy AL and Clarke IC (1981) UCLA anatomic total shoulder arthroplasty. *Clinical Orthopaedics and Related Research* **155** 7–20.

Badley EM, Wagstaff S and Wood PHN (1984) Measures of functional ability (disability) in arthritis in relation to impairment of range of joint movement. *Annals of the Rheumatic Diseases* **43** 563–569.

Barrett WP, Franklin JL, Jackins SE, Wyss CR and Matsen FA III (1987) Total shoulder arthroplasty. *Journal of Bone and Joint Surgery* **69A** 865–872.

Beddow FH (ed.) (1988) *Surgical Management of Rheumatoid Arthritis*. London: Wright.

Bodey WN and Yeoman PM (1983) Prosthetic arthroplasty of the shoulder. *Acta Orthopaedica Scandinavica* **54** 900–903.

Brenner BC, Ferlic DC, Clayton ML and Dennis DA (1989) Survivorship of total shoulder arthroplasty. *Journal of Bone and Joint Surgery* **71A** 1289–1296.

Clayton ML, Ferlic DC and Jeffers PD (1982) Prosthetic arthroplasties of the shoulder. *Clinical Orthopaedics and Related Research* **164** 184–191.

Cofield RH (1984) Total shoulder arthroplasty with the Neer prosthesis. *Journal of Bone and Joint Surgery* **66A** 899–906.

Coughlin MJ, Morris JM and West WF (1979) The semiconstrained shoulder arthroplasty. *Journal of Bone and Joint Surgery* **61A** 574–581.

Crossan JF and Vallance R (1982) The shoulder joint in rheumatoid arthritis. In *Shoulder Surgery* (I Bayley and L Kessel, eds), pp. 131–138. Berlin: Springer.

Dijkstra J, Dijkstra MD and Klundert WVD (1985) Rheumatoid arthritis of the shoulder. Description and standard radiographs. *Fortschritte auf dem Gebiete der Röntgenstrahlen und der Nuklearmedizin* **142** 179–185.

Gristina AG and Webb L (1982) The trispherical total shoulder prosthesis. In *Symposium on Total Joint Replacement of the Upper Extremity* (AE Inglis, ed.) St Louis: Mosby 49–55.

Gschwend N (1980) *Surgical Treatment of Rheumatoid Arthritis*. Philadelphia: Saunders.

Gschwend N and Bischof A (1991) Clinical experiences in arthroplasty according to Neer. *Rheumatology* **4** 135–143.

Hawkins RJ, Bell RH and Jallay B (1989) Total shoulder arthroplasty. *Clinical Orthopaedics and Related Research* **242** 188–194.

Jónsson E (1988) Surgery of the rheumatoid shoulder. Thesis, University of Lund, Sweden.

Jónsson E, Egund N, Kelly IG, Rydholm U and Lidgren L (1986) Cup arthroplasty of the rheumatoid shoulder. *Acta Orthopaedica Scandinavica* **57** 542–546.

Kelly IG (1990a) Surgery of the rheumatoid shoulder. In *The Surgical Management of Rheumatic Diseases* (IG Kelly ed.). Heberden Supplement, *Annals of the Rheumatic Diseases*. pp. 824–829. London: British Medical Association.

Kelly IG (1990b) Shoulder replacement in rheumatoid arthritis. In *Surgery of the Shoulder* (M Post, BF Murray and RJ Hawkins eds) pp. 305–307. St Louis: Mosby.

Kelly IG, Foster RS and Fisher WD (1987) Neer total shoulder replacement in rheumatoid arthritis. *Journal of Bone and Joint Surgery* **69b** 723–736.

Kessel L and Bayley I (1979) Prosthetic replacement of the shoulder: preliminary communication. *Journal of the Royal Society of Medicine* **72** 748–752.

Larsen A, Dale K and Eek M (1977) Radiographic evaluation of rheumatoid arthritis and related conditions by standard reference films. *Acta Radiologica; Diagnosis* **18** 481–491.

Lettin AWF, Copeland SA and Scales J (1982) The Stanmore total shoulder replacement. *Journal of Bone and Joint Surgery* **64B** 47–51.

Marmor L (1977) Hemiarthroplasty for the rheumatoid shoulder joint. *Clinical Orthopaedics and Related Research* **122** 201–203.

Neer CS II (1955) Articular replacement for the humeral head. *Journal of Bone and Joint Surgery* **37A** 215–228.

Neer CS II (1974) Replacement arthroplasty for glenohumeral osteoarthritis. *Journal of Bone and Joint Surgery* **56A** 1–13.

Neer CS II, Watson KC and Stanton FJ (1982) Recent experience in total shoulder arthroplasty. *Journal of Bone and Joint Surgery* **64A** 319–337.

Neer CS II (1990) *Shoulder Reconstruction*. Philadelphia: Saunders.

Pahle JA and Kvarnes L (1985) Shoulder replacement arthroplasty. *Annales Chirurgiae et Gynaecologiae* **74** (Suppl. 198) 85–89.

Petersson CJ (1986) Painful shoulders in patients with rheumatoid arthritis. *Scandinavian Journal of Rheumatology* **15** 275–279.

Poss R, Maloney JF, Ewald FC et al (1984) Six to eleven year results of total hip arthroplasty in rheumatoid arthritis. *Clinical Orthopaedics and Related Research* **182** 109–116.

Post M and Jablon M (1983) Constrained total shoulder arthroplasty. *Clinical Orthopaedics and Related Research* **173** 109–116.

Post M, Haskell SS and Jablon M (1980) Total shoulder replacement with a constrained prosthesis. *Journal of Bone and Joint Surgery* **62A** 327–335.

Roper BA, Paterson JMH and Day WM (1990) The Roper–Day total shoulder replacement. *Journal of Bone and Joint Surgery* **72B** 694–697.

Sledge CB, Kozinn SC, Thornhill TS and Barrett WP (1989) Total shoulder arthroplasty in rheumatoid arthritis. In *Rheumatoid Arthritis Surgery of the Shoulder* (AWF Lettin and C Petersson, eds), pp. 95–102. Basel: Karger.

Steffee AD and Moore RW (1984) Hemi-resurfacing arthroplasty of the shoulder. *Contemporary Orthopaedics* **9** 51–59.

Steinbrocker O, Traeger CH and Batterman RC (1949) Therapeutic criteria in rheumatoid arthritis. *JAMA* **140** 659–662.

Tibrewal SB, Grant KA and Goodfellow JM (1984) The radiolucent zone beneath the tibial component of the Oxford meniscal knee. *Journal of Bone and Joint Surgery* **66B** 523–528.

Varian JPW (1980) Interposition Silastic cup arthroplasty of the shoulder. *Journal of Bone and Joint Surgery* **62B** 116–117.

6

Physiotherapy after unconstrained shoulder replacement

Dorcas Damrel

A correct and carefully graduated treatment regimen is essential to gain a good functional outcome from total shoulder replacement. In many patients the arthritic pain rather than the loss of movement is the major reason for the reduced function of the arm before operation. Once the shoulder pain is relieved by arthroplasty the function of the limb is always improved, even though there may not be a great increase in joint range.

Postoperative physiotherapy is often painful and we have found that patients will co-operate more readily with a potentially painful treatment regimen if the reason for the therapy and the aims of the treatment are explained and they understand the treatment programme. The physiotherapist plays an essential part in this.

The patient's progress is assessed regularly by the physiotherapist, with the joint range, muscle power and limb function being recorded.

Treatment aims

General aims for the patient:

1 To prevent immediate postoperative respiratory and circulatory complications.
2 To aid in the control of postoperative pain.

Specific aims for the shoulder:

3 To maintain, and if possible to increase, the preoperative range of movement.
4 To restore the correct scapulohumeral pattern of movement.

5 To increase the strength of the shoulder musculature.
6 To restore the functional use of the arm.

Preoperative patient management

Before surgery the patient should be fully assessed by the team physiotherapist, with a detailed assessment of the shoulder to be operated on, including range of movement, muscle power, pain and function. Assessment of the elbow and hand is also necessary as the function of the shoulder and arm as a whole may well be affected by the condition of the other joints of the limb.

The operative procedure and postoperative regimen should be explained to the patient before surgery, and also the position of and reason for any wound drains. If an abduction wedge or splint is used postoperatively, this is shown to the patient and its position is demonstrated.

If a written explanation of the postoperative exercise regimen is available this can be given to the patient during the discussion of the rehabilitation programme. The patient is also seen by the occupational therapist who will provide advice about daily living aids that are available, and other functional support.

If the patient needs surgery because of recent trauma a full preoperative assessment will not be possible. The timing of the postoperative regimen will be altered as a result of the effect of the trauma on the rotator cuff. A tear of the rotator cuff which necessitates repair at surgery will also slow down the rehabilitation. The management of these patients is discussed at the end of this chapter.

Postoperative patient management

After surgery, the rehabilitation programme is divided into three stages:

- Early – the first 48 hours after surgery.
- Intermediate – from 3 to 21 days after surgery.
- Late – from 21 days after surgery.

Dr Charles Neer II from New York has been a major influence on shoulder joint replacement and rehabilitation and many of the rehabilitation methods we use are based on his own physiotherapy regimen.

Early – the first 48 hours

The patient will return from the operating theatre with the affected arm in either an abduction wedge or splint (Figure 6.1) or in a sling (Figure 6.2). Postoperative aftercare, consisting of breathing exercises and chest care, active and active assisted elbow flexion and extension, forearm pronation and supination and hand exercises, are practised as a routine. Correct positioning of the abduction splint or sling is essential to support the limb, to ensure

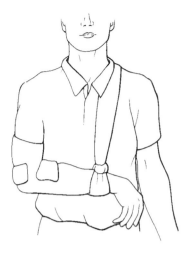

Figure 6.2 The sling.

the patient's comfort and to prevent injury to the ulnar nerve.

Adequate analgesic cover should be provided either systemically or locally. Local analgesia is very satisfactorily provided via an 'epidural' catheter, with a bacterial filter, placed in the subacromial space at operation. This has been found to reduce the need for strong systemic analgesia, with its accompanying side-effects. At our shoulder and elbow unit at Nottingham City Hospital bupivacaine (Marcain), 10 ml 0.25% given 4-hourly locally through the catheter, is used with good effect.

The shoulder is left at rest during this stage. Neck and shoulder girdle posture is corrected and the patients are encouraged to get up and about as much as possible, but this depends on their general condition.

Intermediate – from 3–21 days after surgery

This is the most important stage in the rehabilitation process. During this time movement in all planes is restored or increased, leading to improved shoulder function. If a good range of movement is not achieved by 3 weeks after operation, the shoulder is likely to remain stiff as it is rare to gain much more range after this time. It must be emphasized that the range of movement will be passive. Active movement can take much longer to regain.

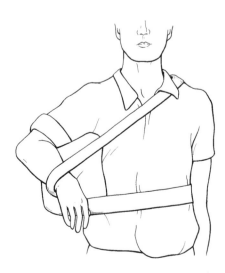

Figure 6.1 The abduction wedge.

Movements of the glenohumeral joint are started 3 days after surgery when the wound drains have been removed. The abduction splint or sling is removed, support of the limb being maintained for the patient's comfort and confidence. The shoulder is taken through an arc of movement which is kept within the patient's pain tolerance level. If the movement is painful, relaxation of the shoulder musculature is difficult and mobilization will be delayed and less satisfactory.

There are several treatment modalities available to the physiotherapist to provide relief of pain. These include:

- Direct heat or cold therapy
- Transcutaneous nerve stimulation
- Pulsed electromagnetic energy
- Interferential.

Active bilateral scapular depression, elevation, protraction and retraction are practised, concentrating particularly on retraction and depression. Shoulder and neck posture continue to be corrected as necessary. Exercises for the elbow and hand are continued to avoid stiffness, especially if there has been extensive bruising of the soft tissues.

During the first 10 days after surgery all movements of the glenohumeral joint should be passive to avoid excessive strain on the recently repaired tissues.

Elevation through flexion, external rotation and internal rotation are the most important functional movements of the shoulder and these are the movements which have most importance during rehabilitation. The exercises are practised 2–3 times a day in sessions lasting between 5 and 15 minutes, depending on the patient's tolerance. Exercises should be supervised by the therapist for the first few days and thereafter they can then be supervised by members of the nursing staff who have been trained by the physiotherapist. This is particularly valuable for treatment over weekends and provides continuity of treatment for the patient. Liaison between the physiotherapy and nursing staff is extremely important in the total care of the patient.

3 days after surgery

Passive flexion by therapist

The patient lies supine and the therapist supports the operated limb with his or her hands. The therapist then lifts the patient's arm into elevation through flexion, increasing the range as the patient's pain allows. Care should be taken to maintain relaxation of the patient's muscles during the exercises.

Passive flexion prone lying (Figure 6.3)

Some patients will not be able to achieve this position, but for those who can it is a useful method of achieving passive shoulder flexion with depression of the shoulder girdle. The weight of the limb gives gentle traction which will assist muscle relaxation. The therapist can also manually stabilize the scapula if necessary, and pendulum exercises can be practised in this position.

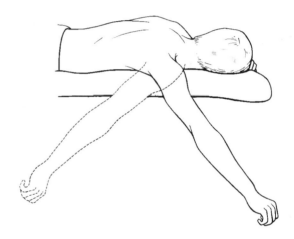

Figure 6.3 Pendular exercises in prone lying. In this position it is easy for the therapist to stabilize the scapula.

Passive external rotation by therapist

This is practised with the patient lying in the supine position. The elbow is flexed to 90° with the arm lying by the patient's side. External rotation is achieved by gently bringing the patient's hand away from the body.

Passive external rotation by patient (Figure 6.4)

A stick is used to achieve passive external rotation of the operated arm by controlled movement of the other arm. It is important to ensure that the elbow is kept into the side during these exercises, otherwise the end result will be abduction rather than external rotation.

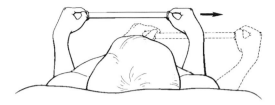

Figure 6.4 Passive external rotation. The elbow can be supported on a rolled towel or similar soft pad for comfort.

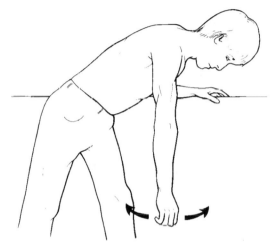

Figure 6.5 Pendulum exercise. This can be performed either sitting or standing. Relaxation of the arm is essential.

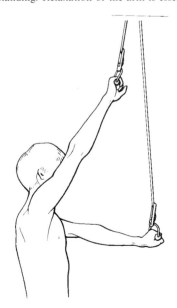

Figure 6.6 Pulley exercise. Passive elevation of the operated arm is achieved by downward pressure of the unoperated arm. Compensatory back extension should be avoided.

Pendulum exercise (Figure 6.5)

The patient leans forward resting the unoperated limb on the back of an upholstered chair or other comfortable support and allowing the operated arm to hang relaxed. Small-range circling movements of the arm are started, the circumference gradually increasing as the mobility and confidence of the patient increases, and as discomfort reduces. Clockwise circles are carried out with the arm in internal rotation, i.e. with the palm facing backwards.

Pulley exercise (Figure 6.6)

The patient can stand or sit to do this exercise. The unoperated arm provides the downward pull on one of the handles to achieve elevation for the operated arm holding the other handle. The patient's posture should be watched and corrected as necessary during this exercise. Both back extension and scapular elevation with rotation will occur if the patient is not trained to adopt a normal position during this exercise.

Passive extension (Figure 6.7)

This exercise can be done either standing or while sitting on a stool. A stick is held between

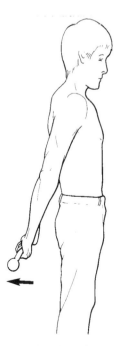

Figure 6.7 Passive extension. Scapular protraction and elevation should be avoided when performing this exercise.

the hands behind the back and the unoperated arm provides the power to aid extension at the glenohumeral joint.

The exercise sessions should be short (about 5–10 minutes) to avoid causing excessive pain, and exercises should be practised 2–3 times a day. The arm is rested on an abduction splint or in a sling at other times.

10 days after surgery

Assisted exercises to gain rotation range are started on the 10th day after operation, as are isometric exercises to strengthen the rotator cuff and deltoid muscles. Isometric exercises are practised to maintain and increase muscle tone. No movement is allowed at the glenohumeral joint during isometric exercises.

In our experience isometric exercises are safe and when carried out under supervision are not associated with disruption of the greater tuberosity osteotomy or subscapularis repair. However, if the subscapularis repair is tenuous, or the bone of the tuberosities is excessively soft or osteoporotic, isometric exercises may be delayed, *at the surgeon's discretion*, for up to 3 weeks after surgery.

The number of daily exercise sessions should be gradually increased over the following 10 days as the patient's pain level reduces and as the power and confidence in the arm improves. The exercise sessions should remain short (5–15 minutes each), to prevent undue fatigue, but the number of sessions can be increased to five or six.

Assisted exercises (from 10 days after surgery)

Assisted external rotation and flexion (Figure 6.8)

This is practised lying supine. The patient holds the wrist of the operated arm with the other hand and lifts the arm upward over the head. The hands are then taken to the back of the neck and the elbows pushed out to the sides to increase the range of external rotation in abduction.

Assisted internal rotation

Method A (Figure 6.9a) This is practised either standing or sitting on a stool. The patient

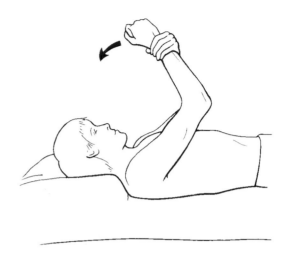

Figure 6.8 Assisted external rotation and flexion. Re-education of the correct scapulothoracic and scapulo-humeral rhythm should be continued during this exercise. The handgrip changes from the unoperated hand clasping the wrist of the operated arm during the flexion phase to fingers linked during the external rotation phase as the hands pass under the head.

holds the wrist of the operated arm with the other hand with hands behind the back and slides the hands up and down the back.
Method B (Figure 6.9b) If it is not possible to get the hands behind the back, possibly due to limited internal rotation of the unoperated arm, a strap can be looped around the wrists and used to assist internal rotation of the operated arm.

Isometric exercises (from 10 days after surgery)

Isometric external rotation

Method A (Figure 6.10a) The patient lies with the operated arm resting on the bed and held close to the body with the elbow flexed to 90°. The other hand is placed on the dorsum of the wrist of the operated arm and resists attempted outward rotation at the shoulder.
Method B (Figure 6.10b) The patient lies with both arms resting on the bed with elbows flexed to 90°. A strap is looped around both wrists and adjusted so that the forearms are vertical and parallel to each other. External rotation of the operated arm is resisted by the resistance from the other arm.

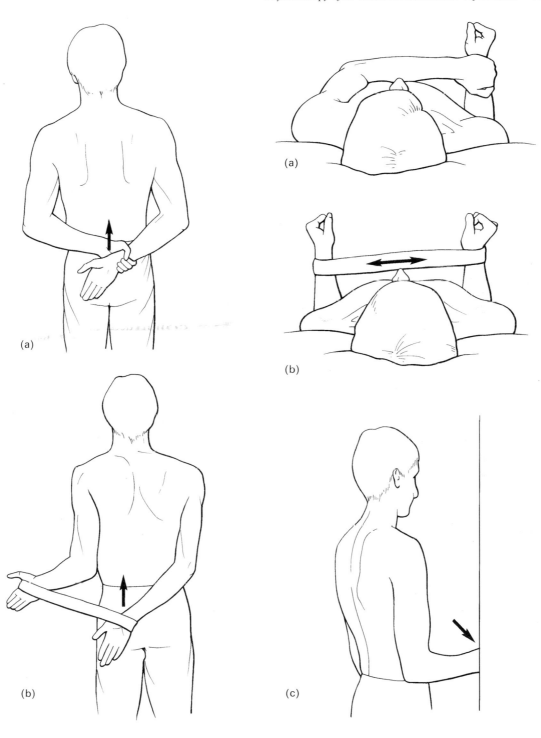

Figure 6.9 Assisted internal rotation. (a) Method A is used when the unoperated arm and hand are mobile and strong and able to reach the other arm behind the back.
(b) Method B is used if there is limited function in the unoperated arm, or if the patient finds this method more comfortable.

Figure 6.10 Isometric external rotation. (a) Method A is used when the operated arm and hand are mobile and strong and able to maintain a steady grip and position.
(b) Method B is used when there is limited function of the unoperated arm, or if the patient finds it more comfortable.

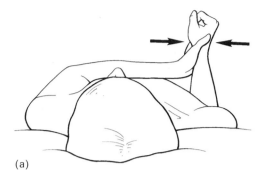

(a)

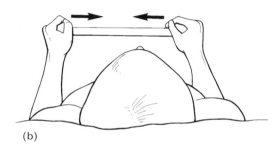

(b)

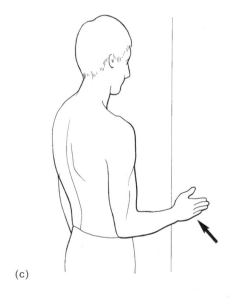

(c)

Figure 6.11 Isometric internal rotation. (a) Method A is used when the unoperated arm and hand are mobile and strong and able to maintain a steady grip and position. (b) Method B is used when there is limited function of the unoperated arm, or if the patient finds it more comfortable. (c) Method C a soft pad can be placed between the wall and the hand for comfort.

Method C (Figure 6.10c)   The patient stands with arm by the side and the elbow flexed to 90°. The dorsum of the hand is placed against a flat surface, such as a wall or door jamb, and the hand is pushed against it. Padding may be placed between the hand and the wall for comfort.

With these exercises care should always be taken to ensure that the position of the upper arm is correctly maintained in contact with the body to prevent abduction rather than isometric external rotation taking place.

Isometric internal rotation

Method A (Figure 6.11a)   The patient lies with the operated arm resting on the bed and held close to the body with the elbow flexed to 90°. The good hand is placed on the flexor aspect of the wrist of the operated arm. The unoperated arm resists and prevents internal rotation of the operated arm.

Method B (Figure 6.11b)   The patient lies with both arms resting on the bed with the elbows flexed to 90°. The patient holds a short stick with padded ends between the hands. The stick should be of a length to allow the patient's forearms to be parallel to each other, and should be padded, particularly at its ends, to enable the patient to hold it easily and comfortably. The patient then attempts to push the hands together against the stick by contraction of the shoulder internal rotators.

Method C (Figure 6.11c)   The patient stands with the arm by the side and the elbow flexed to 90°. Positioning is as for isometric external rotation but with the palm of the hand against a wall or door jamb. The patient then attempts to bring the palm towards the body by pushing against the wall.

Isometric abduction (Figure 6.12)

The patient stands with the operated arm against a wall or other flat surface with the elbow flexed to 90°. Abduction is attempted by pushing the elbow against the wall. The patient should not allow the shoulder girdle to elevate, and this is aided by the patient attempting to push the elbow downwards as well as away from the body.

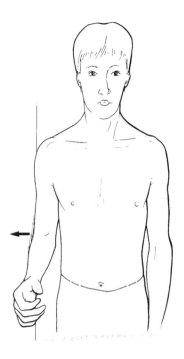

Figure 6.12 Isometric abduction. Correct positioning and stability of the scapula should be maintained so that the glenohumeral abductors (rather than scapular elevators) are contracted.

Isometric extension

Method A (Figure 6.13a)   The patient lies with both arms resting on the bed with the elbows flexed to 90°. The elbows are then pushed downwards and backwards into the bed. Doing the exercise bilaterally prevents rotation of the patient towards the operated limb and aids shoulder girdle retraction.

Method B (Figure 6.13b)   The patient stands with the back to the wall, the arms by the sides and the elbows flexed to 90°. The elbows are pushed backwards against the wall. Doing the exercises bilaterally prevents rotation of the patient towards the operated limb and aids shoulder girdle retraction.

14 days after surgery

Treatment at this stage is designed to maintain and increase the power in the deltoid muscle. Active abduction and flexion can be commenced, using suspension if the muscles are very weak. This method can also be used to achieve correct shoulder girdle synchrony. The exercises are practised initially with a short

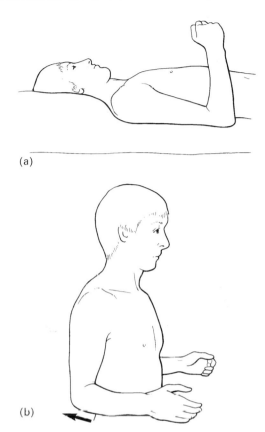

Figure 6.13 Isometric extension. It is easier for the therapist to correct scapular position in method A (a).

lever, i.e. with the elbow flexed, progressing to a long lever, i.e. with the elbow extended, when muscle power is adequate.

The patient should continue to practise a selection of the earlier exercises. If an abduction splint or wedge has been used, it can now be discarded and an arm sling used when necessary for comfort only.

The patient should now be encouraged to use the arm for normal daily activities such as bathing, dressing and eating, but should be dissuaded from prolonged use of the arm or stressing the shoulder in activities such as lifting or pushing heavy doors.

Hydrotherapy can be a useful adjunct to the treatment routine if the patient's wound is healed and his or her general condition allows it. An occlusive dressing, such as Opsite, can be used over the wound as additional protection. The heat of the hydrotherapy pool aids muscle relaxation and reduces pain, and the buoyancy assists active exercises.

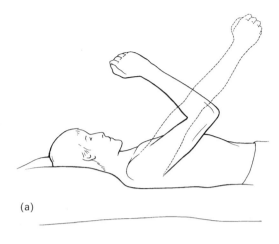

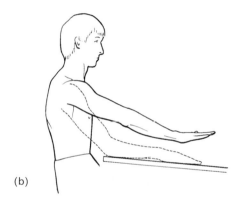

Figure 6.14 Active flexion. (a) Method A: progression is made as glenohumeral control improves. (b) Method B increases the loading on the muscles.

Active flexion

Method A (Figure 6.14a)   This is performed lying with the arm by the side and the elbow flexed to 90°. The arm is lifted over the head and gradually lowered in stages through various points in the range of movement. As muscle power increases the exercise is practised with the elbow extended.

Method B (Figure 6.14b)   This is practised sitting at a table or flat-topped desk. The hand is placed on the surface and slid forwards by increasing the flexion range at the glenohumeral joint, keeping the shoulder girdle protracted and depressed. The patient should be discouraged from lifting the hand off the surface by retracting or elevating the shoulder girdle or by extending the spine.

Late – from 21 days after surgery

Resisted exercises and passive stretching. These exercises are performed to increase muscle power further and improve the range of both active and passive joint movement. Resistance to movement can be supplied by the therapist using techniques such as proprioceptive neuro-muscular facilitation, but the majority of patients carry out their exercise programme themselves using Cliniband or Theraband.

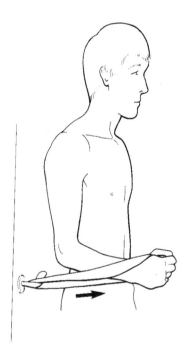

Figure 6.15 Resisted flexion. Movement should just occur at the glenohumeral joint.

Resisted exercises

Flexion (Figure 6.15)

One end of a loop of Cliniband Theraband (exercise rubber) is fixed firmly round a door handle. The patient stands facing away from the door holding the other end of the loop in the hand, with the elbow flexed to 90°. The arm is then pushed forward to stretch the Cliniband. This position is held for up to 5 seconds for each repetition.

Extension (Figure 6.16)

One end of a loop of Cliniband is fixed firmly round a door handle. The patient stands facing

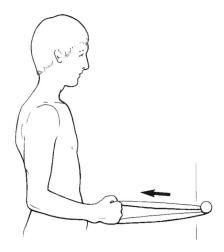

Figure 6.16 Resisted extension. This can be combined with scapular retraction and depression for posture correction.

the door. The arm is then pulled backwards to stretch the Cliniband. This position is held for up to 5 seconds for each repetition.

External rotation (Figure 6.17)

The patient stands or sits with the upper arm by the sides and the elbows bent to 90°. The Cliniband is looped around the wrists and stretched by the patient moving the hands apart while keeping the elbows close to the sides. This position is held for up to 5 seconds for each repetition.

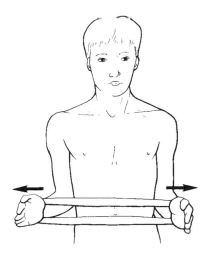

Figure 6.17 Resisted external rotation. The shoulder should not abduct or extend during this exercise. It can be combined with scapular retraction and depression for posture correction.

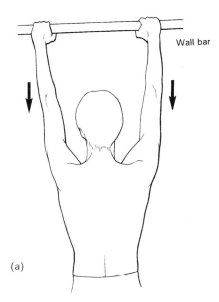

(a)

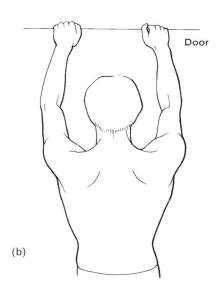

(b)

Figure 6.18 Flexion stretching. The shoulder should be allowed to stretch gently and gradually into increased flexion. The patient should be discouraged from pulling up on the hands.

Stretching

Flexion

Method A (Figure 6.18a) This method uses wall bars so is usually only possible when the patient attends the physiotherapy department.

The operated arm is assisted up into flexion using the other hand and both hands are hooked over the highest wall bars the patient can reach. The patient then bends the knees slightly to increase shoulder flexion.

Method B (Figure 6.18b)   The patient stands facing a door. The operated arm is assisted up into flexion by the other hand until both hands can be hooked over the top of the door. The patient then bends the knees slightly to stretch the shoulder and increase shoulder flexion. The patient may need to stand on a stool to reach the top of the door, so the age and general fitness of the patient should be taken into consideration before attempting this exercise.

If this exercise is not possible, an alternative is to obtain stretching and passive flexion by hooking the fingers over a stair, if there is an open staircase, or else by using a high cupboard drawer, shelf or cupboard door (providing it is firm and secure).

External rotation (Figure 6.19)

The patient stands in a doorway with the elbow flexed to 90° and held close to the body. The hand is placed on the door jamb and the body is slowly turned away from it, pushing the shoulder into external rotation. The side of a cupboard or a wall can also be used for this exercise.

Internal rotation (Figure 6.20)

The patient places a small towel lengthways over the unoperated shoulder. One end is grasped behind the back by the hand of the operated arm and the other end is held in front of the body by the good hand. The good hand is then moved forwards and downwards pulling the operated arm up the back and increasing internal rotation.

Hospital discharge

The patient is usually discharged from hospital after about 3 weeks of inpatient rehabilitation. If patients live near the hospital and can attend regularly as outpatients they may be discharged earlier.

Before being discharged, the patient will normally be seen and assessed by an occupational therapist and medical social worker, as

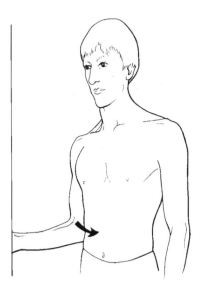

Figure 6.19 External rotation stretching. If the shoulder tends to go into extension during this exercise, the elbow can be supported by the unoperated hand. The stretch should be gentle and controlled.

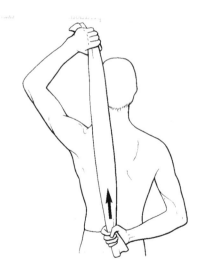

Figure 6.20 Internal rotation stretching. The stretch should be gentle and controlled, with the dorsum of the hand kept against the back and good body posture maintained.

necessary. Home support services, such as a home help or a district nurse, are organized as required.

The patient will require exercise equipment at home. This will include a set of pulleys, a short padded stick (or a walking stick) and a loop of

Cliniband. Patients should continue to practise their exercises regularly at home for at least 6 months. They usually find that they continue to increase their strength for up to 6 months after surgery and feel that they stiffen up if they miss out the joint mobility exercises.

Most patients would *not* need outpatient physiotherapy, but attendance once a week for assessment of progress until the 6-week stage is useful for a few. If it is found that the patient is losing range or having problems with the exercise regimen a short course of more frequent treatment can then be organized.

At 6 weeks after surgery the patient should be able to:

- Put the hand to the back of the neck.
- Put the hand behind the back.
- Flex the arm forwards to 90° with the elbow extended.

Resuming household tasks or employment depends greatly on the patient's general condition. The following are our guidelines for a patient with an intact rotator cuff and stable tuberosity osteotomy after operation.

Housework:	vacuuming 4 weeks
	ironing 4 weeks
Hobbies:	swimming 4 weeks
	gentle gardening, e.g. hand weeding and light planting, 6 weeks minimum
Driving a car:	6 weeks minimum
Work:	sedentary 6 weeks
	more active 12 weeks
	heavy up to 16 weeks

In certain circumstances the patient will not be able to return to their previous occupation and referral to a disablement resettlement officer may be necessary.

Shoulder replacement after trauma and/or associated with a rotator cuff repair

In these patients any stress on the rotator cuff must be delayed until adequate healing of both the bone and the soft tissues has taken place. If a repair of an extensive rotator cuff tear has been carried out the cuff should be protected during rehabilitation for up to 6 weeks. We recommend that the limb is splinted in an abduction splint for at least 3 weeks to protect the healing tissues. Passive glenohumeral movement into elevation should be practised during this period to prevent joint stiffness and tissue adhesions. The shoulder is gradually mobilized within the patient's pain tolerance. If practicable, the patient may be discharged home once a range of at least 120° of elevation has been regained. The patient's partner should be taught how to carry out the passive elevation exercises before the patient's discharge, and the physiotherapist will ensure that the partner is confident in handling the patient's arm and in looking after any splintage before the patient leaves hospital.

If the abduction splint is retained for 6 weeks, the patient will normally be discharged home at 2 weeks and readmitted at 6 weeks for continuation of the rehabilitation programme. The arm is then gradually brought back to the side by adjusting the splint over a period of 48 hours. This often causes some aching in the arm. Isometric, active and finally strengthening exercises are then started, as tolerated by the patient. Up to 1 week in hospital will be required for this.

We have found that the rehabilitation of patients with joint replacement after recent trauma normally takes longer. Younger patients often need a more extended period of outpatient rehabilitation as their aims and expectations are for a near normal shoulder.

Conclusion

Pain relief is the main aim of shoulder replacement. A satisfactory improvement in function can be achieved if the joint pain is relieved, even if there is not a great increase in joint range, but the condition of the other joints of the limb must be taken into account before setting the postoperative goals. Some patients will continue functional improvement for up to a year after surgery before reaching a plateau, but the most important period for therapy is during the first 3 weeks postoperatively. The full co-operation of the patient is essential in order to obtain the maximum benefit from these joint replacement procedures – much more so than for knee or hip replacement.

Further reading

Neer CS (1982) Arthroplasty of the shoulder: Neer technique. 3M surgical protocol manual. Loughborough: 3M Health Care Ltd.

Newton I and Homfray C (1985) The total shoulder replacement: management and treatment. *Journal of the Association of Orthopaedic Chartered Physiotherapists* **Oct.** 5–9.

7

Revision shoulder replacement and rotator cuff problems

W. Angus Wallace

Charles Neer II has pioneered shoulder replacement surgery in the USA and shoulder arthroplasty is now becoming increasing popular in Europe. Total shoulder replacement using the Neer II components began in 1974 (Neer, Watson and Stanton, 1982) – only 23 years ago – and these implants (or similar designs) remain the most commonly used worldwide. With the resulting increased surgical activity more patients are presenting with problems related to their prosthesis and some will require revision surgery. The surgeon has a duty to clearly identify why the patient does not have a good result from the previous shoulder replacement operation and if there is a remediable cause for the patient's dissatisfaction with the shoulder. The importance of the soft tissues and surrounding anatomy in producing a normally functioning shoulder cannot be over emphasized. A 'minor soft tissue or bony procedure' carried out after the main shoulder joint replacement operation is sometimes necessary to obtain an optimal result so it is difficult to define accurately what is a 'revision' operation.

A revision procedure is defined here as: 'any further surgical procedure carried out on the same shoulder of a patient who has previously been treated with an arthroplasty to that shoulder'. Such revision procedures might therefore include complications from the surgical approach, from rotator cuff deficiency and from post-operative displacement of the tuberosities, as well as the more widely recognized indications for revision: loosening, infection and wear of the components.

Revision rates

Revision rates for shoulder hemiarthroplasty and total shoulder replacement are low, partly because most surgeons are reluctant to offer revision surgery as it is difficult and partly because the outcome from revision operations is difficult to predict. Certain groups of patients have been identified as more commonly having poor results after shoulder arthroplasty:

- Patients with rheumatoid arthritis with rotator cuff defects (Hirst and Wallace, 1987; Thomas, Amstutz and Cracchiolo, 1991).
- Patients treated late after fracture mal union or post-traumatic arthritis.
- Patients in whom osteotomy of the greater tuberosity was performed at the time of arthroplasty.

Cofield and Edgerton (1990) have reviewed the literature on the complications following shoulder replacement published between 1972 and 1988. Table 7.1 summarizes these papers.

From personal experience of over 300 arthroplasties carried out between 1983 and 1993, the author believes the figures in Table 7.1 underestimate the complication rate from primary shoulder arthroplasty. Each complication will be reviewed in the light of the author's personal experience from these 300 primary arthroplasties. Fifty-three shoulders have required revision surgery – a revision rate of 18%. As some of these patients have had more than

Table 7.1 Reported complications of shoulder arthroplasty (From Cofield and Edgerton, 1990)

Complication	Unconstrained TSR (%)	Constrained TSR (%)	Hemiarthroplasty (%)
Glenoid loosening	4.7 (0–36)	11.8 (0–25)	—
Humeral loosening	0.4 (0–6.9)	1.0 (0–7.7)	—
Subluxation	0.9 (0–12.5)	—	0
Dislocation	2.7 (0–18.2)	9.4 (6–16.7)	1.7 (2–6.6)
Rotator cuff tear	2.2 (0–16.6)	0	2.7 (2–11.5)
Infection	0.5 (0–3.9)	2.9 (0–15.4)	0
Nerve injury	0.5 (0–2)	0	0.4 (0–2)

Percentages are averages; values in parentheses are ranges. TSR, total shoulder replacement.

one revision operation, the total number of revision operations was 68.

Glenoid loosening (Figure 7.1)

One hundred and two cemented Neer II glenoids were inserted between 1983 and 1990. Of these, eight have required revision surgery for symptomatic loosening of the glenoid: four in rheumatoid patients, two in Charcot patients and two in patients treated for cuff tear arthropathy. In addition there are a further three patients on the waiting list for surgery because of symptomatic glenoid loosening.

Eighty-six uncemented glenoid components (mainly biomodular) were inserted between 1990 and 1993. Of these only one has required early revision for loosening – a patient who had habitual anterior dislocation! In a second patient the glenoid liner has become detached from the metal porous coated base and this

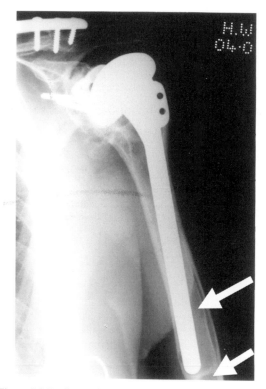

Figure 7.2 Radiograph of a hemiarthroplasty showing humeral component loosening (arrowed).

patient is awaiting surgery to replace the liner – a special problem for the modular components.

Although this series is unfairly biased against the cemented glenoids, which have been in place longer, our experience with porous ingrowth glenoid components indicates they may be associated with less loosening in the long term.

Humeral loosening (Figure 7.2)

Of the 300 shoulder arthroplasties, only three have required revision for symptomatic humeral loosening to date. A further three patients

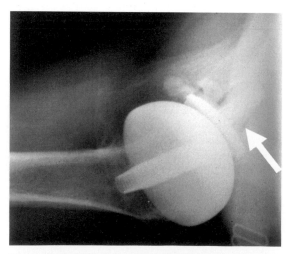

Figure 7.1 Radiograph of a shoulder arthroplasty with obvious glenoid component loosening (arrowed).

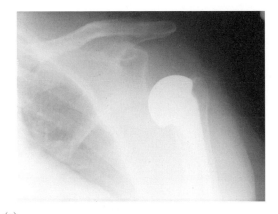

(a)

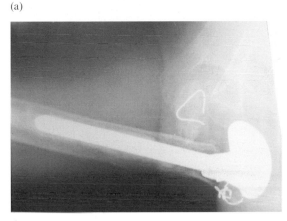

(b)

Figure 7.3 (a) and (b) Anterior subluxation after total shoulder arthroplasty.

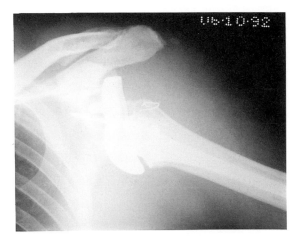

Figure 7.4 Anterior dislocation after shoulder arthroplasty.

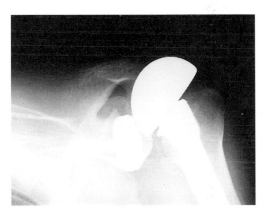

Figure 7.5 Posterior dislocation after shoulder arthroplasty.

are awaiting humeral revision. However, a number of Neer II humeral components inserted without cement have subsided and in these patients the shoulder function has deteriorated, with the return of aching discomfort in the arm. It is recommended that all humeral prostheses which are not specifically designed for uncemented use should be inserted with cement.

Subluxation (Figure 7.3)

This complication is difficult to define because the borderline between a slightly lax shoulder and a shoulder which subluxes is not clear. Approximately six patients with painful subluxation of the shoulder – most commonly due to rotator cuff laxity or deficiency – have been offered revision surgery. Surgical treatment usually involved a soft tissue adjustment such as plication of the rotator cuff, but in some patients extensive revision of the implants was

required in order to obtain the correct balancing of the rotator cuff. Despite careful attention to detail and attempts to balance the rotator cuff correctly, only three of these procedures were successful.

Dislocation (Figures 7.4 and 7.5)

Six patients have required reoperation for dislocation of the shoulder: three for anterior dislocation and three for posterior dislocation. Two of the cases of anterior dislocation occurred due to subscapularis deficiency in rheumatoid patients. In two cases we believe that the anterior dislocation was associated with the abduction splint slipping posteriorly during the postoperative period, thus encouraging the shoulder to dislocate anteriorly – a problem which is avoided with good nursing

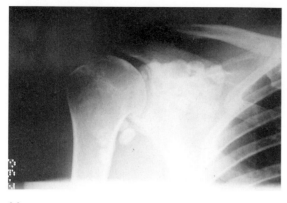

(a)

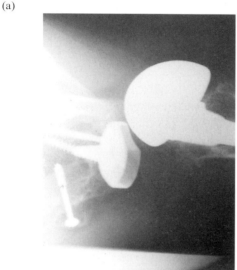

(b)

Figure 7.6 (a) and (b) Osteoarthritis with secondary synovial chondromatosis leading to postarthroplasty posterior dislocation.

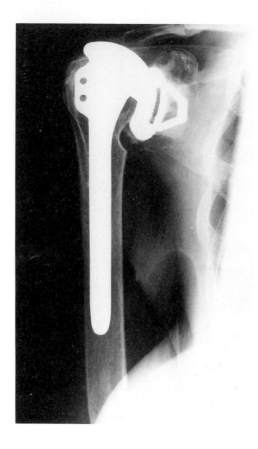

Figure 7.7 A high-riding humeral arthroplasty following a rotator cuff tear. (Note the slightly displaced clavicular osteotomy).

care. Two of the posterior dislocations occurred in patients with osteoarthritis who appeared to have excessive infraspinatus laxity. This occurs either because of a combination of huge osteophytes and preoperative posterior subluxation with posterior glenoid erosion, or because of massive stretching of the infraspinatus related to secondary multiple osteochondromatosis (Figure 7.6). It is important to plicate the infraspinatus and posterior capsule from inside in such cases.

Rotator cuff tears (Figure 7.7)

Seven shoulders in patients with rheumatoid arthritis were revised because of rotator cuff tears. In addition, three patients with rotator cuff arthropathy and two patients with fracture malunions treated with arthroplasty had subsequent cuff tears requiring reoperation. These operations were all difficult and will be discussed later in this chapter.

Infection (Figure 7.8)

In this series of 300 arthroplasties there were only four deep infections, with three of these occurring after revision operations. This gives an infection rate for primary arthroplasty of 0.3% and for revision arthroplasty of around 3–4%. The increased risk of deep infection after a revision operation has occurred despite perioperative antibiotic prophylaxis and the use of a laminar flow clean-air enclosure for almost all primary cases and for every revision operation. Our management of the infected

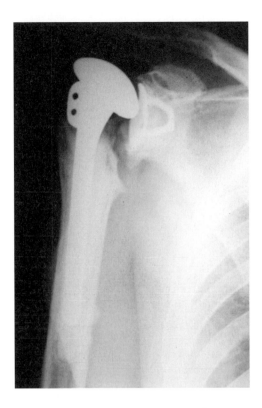

Figure 7.8 Deep infection with loosening and a periosteal reaction.

cases has depended on the type of organism cultured and whether the infection has been adequately controlled before revision surgery. If there was no pus at revision and the previously cultured organism was a staphylococcus, then a one-stage exchange operation was carried out. In two cases the shoulder was treated with an excision arthroplasty with remarkably good results, as shown in Figure 7.9.

Nerve injury

Despite the proximity of the brachial plexus and the large nerves exiting from it, remarkably few nerve injuries have occurred with shoulder arthroplasty operations. Three major nerve injuries were associated with hemiarthroplasty for acute fractures: two axillary and one radial. These were probably operative injuries. In addition there have been at least three temporary axillary nerve palsies after total shoulder arthroplasty. In one case where a one-stage revision operation was being carried

out for infection, the humeral cement was being reamed with a power reamer which perforated the posterior cortex of the bone and destroyed the radial nerve. This was an avoidable complication which the author cites as a good reason for the use of an uncemented humeral stem, revision of which can be done without the risky removal of cement distally in the humeral shaft.

In addition to the above well-recognized indications for revision surgery the author's own series include the following.

Peroperative humeral shaft fractures (Figure 7.10)

Three were identified at the time of the operation and dealt with by using a long humeral stem and cerclage wire. One was unfortunately not picked up until the first postoperative radiograph and the patient had to be taken back to the operating theatre for corrective surgery.

Revision for bony impingement

This is usually secondary to a non-anatomical reconstruction. This complication was remarkably common in this series, with nine cases requiring revision. In five cases the problem appeared to be related to a malunion of the greater tuberosity which was considered acceptable at primary surgery but which appeared to cause impingement postoperatively. In four cases the impingement was felt to have been related to a prominent exostosis from either osteoarthritis or external callus.

Reoperations related to the surgical approach (Figure 7.11)

The author uses a clavicular osteotomy (as described below) for over 180% of primary shoulder arthroplasties, as well as for all revision arthroplasties. In this series of 300 arthroplasties a clavicular fracture occurred in association with the clavicular osteotomy on six occasions (3% fracture incidence), requiring intraoperative plating in two cases and a second plating operation postoperatively in four cases. In addition, some patients have been noted to have some deltopectoral muscle deficiency but none has required surgical repair. Two patients

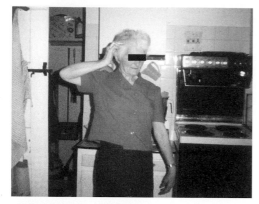

(a)

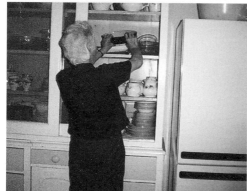

(b)

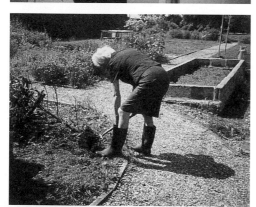

(c)

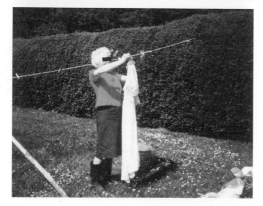

(d)

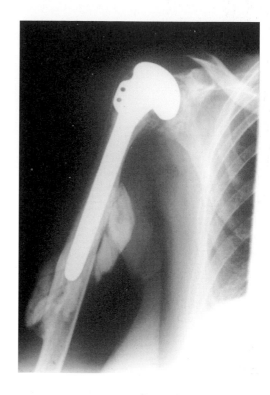

Figure 7.10 A peroperative humeral shaft fracture.

have had late disruptions of muscles: one due to a lesser tuberosity displacement 7 weeks after operation (after the patient had fallen off a bus seat as the bus went round a corner); and one middle third deltoid avulsion from the acromion in a wheelchair user 7 months after an acromioplasty.

Surgical approach for revision shoulder arthroplasty

Revision operations on the shoulder are particularly difficult and a good exposure of the front of the shoulder is required in order to obtain the best results. The modified anterior extensile approach popularized by Redfern, Wallace and Beddow (1989) is recommended as the standard surgical approach for revision surgery. It is also the approach used by the author for over 90% of primary arthroplasty operations.

Figure 7.9 (a)–(d) Functional result 2 years after right shoulder excision arthroplasty for infection.

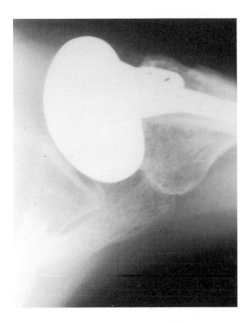

Figure 7.11 Clavicular fracture after clavicular osteotomy.

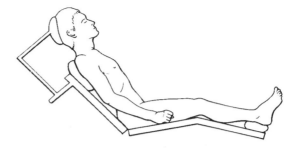

Figure 7.12 The dental chair or astronaut position.

Modified anterior extensile approach (Wallace, 1991)

The patient is positioned in the dental chair or astronaut position, as shown in Figure 7.12. The trunk is tilted upwards at an angle of 45°, thus reducing venous pressure and the risk of bleeding. The scapula is stabilized by placing a 500 ml plastic saline infusion bag under the medial border of the scapula. An incision 10 cm long starts at the level of the clavicle and passes vertically down, across the tip of the coracoid, and distally passes just lateral to the anterior axillary fold (Figure 7.13). The cephalic vein is located (if not previously tied off) in the distal deltopectoral groove and dissected upwards, with ligation of its lateral branches. If bleeding is a problem, the vein may be tied at the top and bottom of its exposed section. The lateral third of the clavicle is now exposed by dissection in the subcutaneous layer (Figure 7.14). The acromioclavicular joint is most easily identified by probing for the joint space with a 21-gauge needle. The periosteum lying over the lateral third of the clavicle is now divided longitudinally, with the retention of the muscular attachments of the deltoid below and trapezius above. Using an oscillating saw with a short narrow blade and cutting downwards, the anterior one-third of the thickness of the lateral third of the

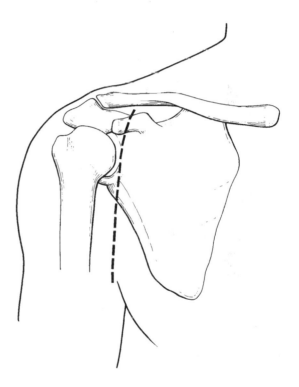

Figure 7.13 The modified anterior extensile approach – skin incision.

clavicle is cut from the main part of the bone. The saw cut is brought anteriorly both medially at the attachment of the deltoid and laterally just before the acromioclavicular joint is reached (Figure 7.15). Care should be taken to produce a smooth curve at the medial end of the cut because any sharp corners will act as stress raisers, with a subsequent risk of clavicle fracture. The whole of the clavicular attachment of deltoid is now attached to the separated bony bar of anterior clavicle which can be

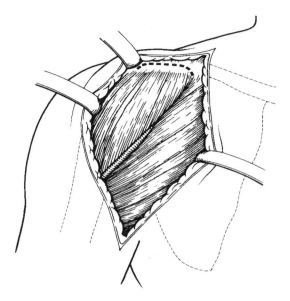

Figure 7.14 Exposure of the lateral third of the clavicle.

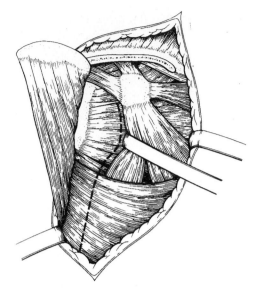

Figure 7.16 The front of the glenohumeral joint area and the coracoacromial ligament exposed after reflecting the osteotomized anterior clavicle with its attached deltoid.

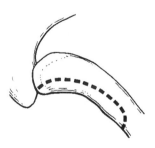

Figure 7.15 The shape of the smooth clavicular osteotomy created using an oscillating saw.

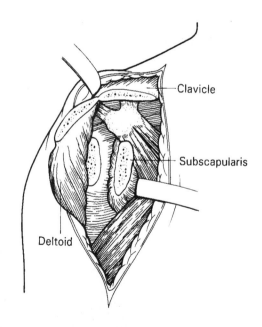

Figure 7.17 Access to the glenohumeral joint is obtained by osteotomizing the lesser tuberosity and externally rotating the arm.

reflected laterally with sharp dissection, as shown in Figure 7.16. The rotator cuff may now be exposed by dividing or excising the coracoacromial ligament. Access to the glenohumeral joint is best obtained by osteotomy of the lesser tuberosity from the humeral head (Figure 7.17). The subscapularis tendon is separated from the supraspinatus tendon along the line of the rotator interval, which is an ill-defined line joining the bicipital groove to the base of the coracoid. Once capsular adhesions are divided the humeral prosthesis is exposed by simply externally rotating the arm gently. The CA ligament may be divided (and later repaired) for an even better access.

Dealing with the implants

If the humeral component is a cemented one-piece component the greater tuberosity area is explored and all the cement and bone proximal

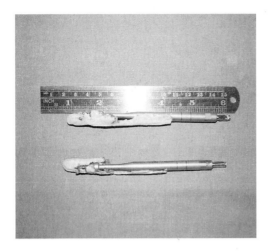

Figure 7.18 Removal of the cement plug using the ultrasonic cement extractor.

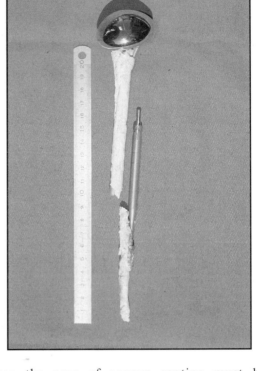

to the lateral fin of the prosthesis is removed. If wire was used to reattach the tuberosities this should now be removed, and once all obvious obstructions to sliding out the humeral component have been dealt with a punch is applied to the undersurface of the humeral head and firmly struck with a hammer. The Neer II components are designed to slide out of cement and it is rare to have a major problem with their removal. On the glenoid side, the glenoid component should be inspected and all soft tissue removed from around the prosthesis–bone interface. The glenoid should now be gently levered to look for movement between the component and bone. If movement is possible, the glenoid component should be removed and replaced. In most cases, as the glenoid component is levered out of the scapula, there is sufficient loss of bone stock for the cement to slip out, but if there is doubt the cement should be broken up with an osteotome before removal by tilting the loose glenoid component, slipping an osteotome along the bone–cement gap and chipping away at the glenoid cement mass.

If a porous coated two-piece uncemented humeral component is being revised first the liner should be removed, then the screws and then the area of porous coating must be identified and mechanical separation of the bone from the implant at the bone ingrowth interface is necessary using either a saw or appropriate osteotomes before attempting to use a punch or an extractor on the prosthesis. For the modular humeral component, the only two reasons for removing the humeral stem would be malposition of the stem – particularly malrotation, or infection. Removal of the biomodular stem is very difficult because of ingrowth into the porous coating; and using an osteotome or an oscillating saw, it is usually necessary to 'dismantle' the proximal humerus from the prosthesis to allow its removal, often leaving an 'exploded' proximal humerus which has to be rebuilt around the new humeral component. The author has experience of removing only three biomodular components and recommends that suitable materials (wire and Dacron tape) are available for reconstruction of the proximal humerus after this procedure. The biomodular instrumentation (including the slide hammer) for removing the humeral component is not ideal and additional instruments, including a Mole wrench (vice grips), are required.

For cemented humeral components, removal

of the humeral cement should not be carried out until the glenoid has been fully prepared for insertion of the new glenoid component to avoid the risk of humeral shaft fracture – a very real risk during revision procedures. Experience with the ultrasonic cement-removing apparatus in four cases has been so satisfactory (Figure 7.18) that the author now feels that this (or similar) equipment is very beneficial for such revision surgery. Our experience has indicated a 40% reduction in the operating time required to remove the cement, and far less risk of fracturing or perforating the humerus.

It is currently the author's practice to revise all shoulder arthroplasties to uncemented or Nottingham total shoulder arthroplasties because of the advantages of improved glenoid fixation, better reattachment of the tuberosities and more adjustable rotator cuff tensioning.

Rotator cuff deficiencies and their management at arthroplasty

Clinical experience in rheumatoid arthritis has highlighted the very real problems associated with the deficient rotator cuff in these patients. Hirst and Wallace (1987) reported a series of 12 patients with rheumatoid arthritis treated with shoulder arthroplasty. Seven patients, all with good intact rotator cuffs at surgery, had excellent or good results, but five patients with cuff tears of 3 cm or more at surgery all had an unsatisfactory result, usually because of loss of function, despite attempts to repair the cuff at operation. A similar experience has been reported by McCoy et al (1989) who had poorer results in seven of the 29 shoulders in their series which had rotator cuff tears. Vahvanen et al (1989) and Thomas et al (1991) have commented that after shoulder arthroplasty up to 50% of rheumatoid patients develop proximal migration of the humeral component at follow-up, indicating 'rotator cuff deficiency' which is usually associated with poor movement, although pain relief is often satisfactory. The author has attempted to improve his own results by ensuring the glenoid component is positioned with a downward tilt of 5–10° in an attempt to reduce upward migration of the humeral component for the biomechanical reasons discussed in Chapter 2.

Two methods have been adopted to deal with

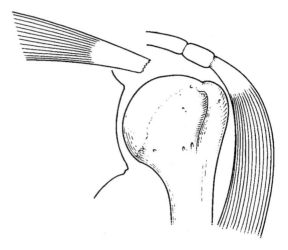

Figure 7.19 The Nottingham (terylene) hood – the rotator cuff tear.

patients with major rotator cuff deficiencies (Wallace, 1990):

1 By reducing the length of the hard tissues (i.e. the humeral head) the gap in the rotator cuff can be reduced.
2 By reinforcing the rotator cuff repair with an artificial 'Nottingham hood' the remaining poor quality tendon tissue can at least be fixed to a secure anchoring point.

The principles behind this procedure are summarized in Figures 7.19–7.21. Unfortunately the medium-term results from the use of the Nottingham hood in 25 shoulders with a follow-up of 4 years (Wallace, Schippinger and Neumann, 1993) have not been as good as had been hoped. The Nottingham hood has now been modified with a more open weave to allow better soft tissue anchorage; this may provide better results in the future.

Dealing with bone deficiency at primary and revision surgery

Once all components are removed at revision surgery, the next step is to reconstruct the necessary bone stock to allow a satisfactory and solid replacement of both the glenoid and the humeral components. On the glenoid side, the whole of the glenoid must be exposed and inspected. There may be anterior, posterior or central bony deficiency. Central bony deficiency

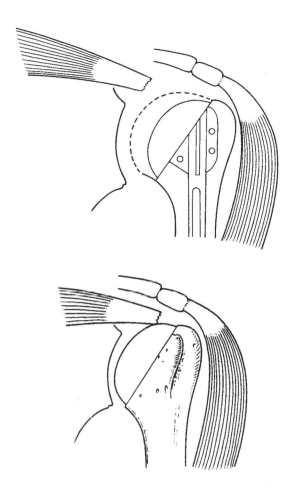

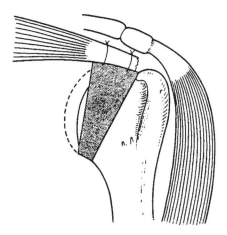

Figure 7.21 Application of the Nottingham hood and reconstruction of the rotator cuff over the top of the hood. Note the hood has been designed as a reinforcement for the cuff, not as a replacement for it.

Figure 7.20 Removal of the humeral head and the insertion of a narrow humeral head to reduce the rotator cuff deficiency.

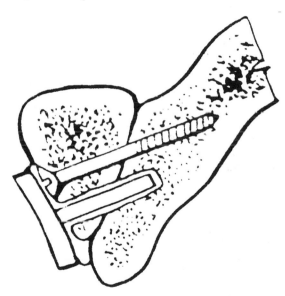

Figure 7.22 A wedge of bone used to correct a posterior glenoid deficiency.

is easiest to deal with – either by using autogenous graft (a block of iliac crest or cancellous chips) or using allograft (a block of morselized bone). Using a revision cemented component is less than ideal because of the difficulty in obtaining a satisfactory interlock with the cement; the author favours the use of a porous backed component which is anchored with deep pitched screws. In cases with anterior or posterior glenoid deficiency a wedge of bone, as shown in Figure 7.22, can be used but this is mechanically not ideal. One method used on two occasions was to split the glenoid vertically with an oscillating saw and lever apart the anterior cortex of the scapular neck from the posterior cortex. A wedge-shaped iliac crest or allograft could then be inserted into the gap and fashioned to recreate a flat glenoid face (Figure

7.23) before applying the selected glenoid component or choosing to use a hemiarthroplasty only. The most difficult case the author has dealt with was a 24-year-old woman with rheumatoid arthritis who had undergone two previous operations: a Varian cup arthroplasty (Figure 7.24), which became fragmented and painful, followed by a Neer II total shoulder replacement in which the glenoid was cemented in a poor position (Figure 7.25). After 2 years the glenoid became loose and painful (Figure

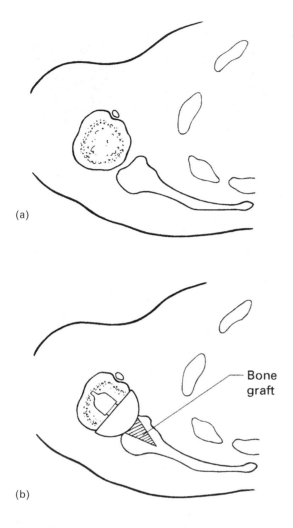

(a)

(b)

— Bone
graft

Figure 7.23 (a) and (b) The glenoid is osteotomized
vertically, the bone graft wedge is inserted into the
separated anterior and posterior cortices and the new 'face'
of the glenoid is recreated.

7.26). At revision the glenoid was found to be
almost completely destroyed but it was possible
to position a block of allograft on the remaining bone and an uncemented biomodular
component could then be anchored on to the
allograft block in an improved position using
two screws (Figure 7.27). At follow-up 36
months later the shoulder was pain free with
active elevation to 120° and a satisfactory
radiological appearance.

On the humeral side bony reconstruction is
easier and the use of cancellous graft to obtain
union of the tuberosities is strongly encour-

aged. It is vital that the whole rotator cuff is
reconstructed and Dacron tape (DuPont, Wil-
mington, DE) used to effect a strong and stable
reconstruction of the tuberosities and the cuff,
has become popular (Figure 7.28), although the
author still regularly used 1.2 mm stainless steel
wire. It is the author's practice to use a
cementless humeral stem but to cement in the
distal stem in revision cases, leaving the
proximal porous coated end to encourage
re-attachment of the tuberosities.

What can be achieved with revision surgery?

The possibility of improving the result from a
shoulder arthroplasty by carrying out a revision
operation should always be considered but the
experienced surgeon knows that before embarking on surgery the following points must be
clear:

- If reoperation is being carried out for pain,
  is the pain the result of a mechanical
  problem? If the pain is related to a past
  nerve injury, as it was in one of the
  author's cases, it will not respond to
  revision surgery.
- Pain presenting after a previously successful shoulder arthroplasty is likely to arise
  from a mechanically loose glenoid component and this is not always obvious on
  radiographs.
- Post-arthroplasty stiffness is very difficult
  to correct with further surgery. These
  shoulders often restiffen despite an intensive post-revision physiotherapy programme.
- The patient must know the risks associated
  with revision surgery (infection 2–4%,
  nerve injury 2–4%, less than 90° of movement in over 50% of cases) but these risks
  are usually worth taking in patients who
  have moderate to severe pain.
- Post-arthroplasty instability is difficult to
  correct and the surgeon must be satisfied
  that the patient's disability fully justifies a
  major revision procedure.

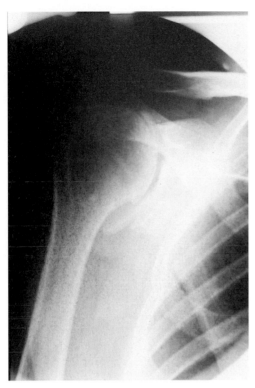

Figure 7.24 A 24-year-old woman with rheumatoid arthritis was treated initially with a Varian cup arthroplasty. Note the fragmentation of the Silastic cup.

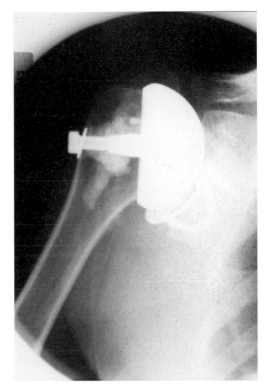

Figure 7.25 Copeland humeral replacement carried out at 28 years old. Note the poor position of the Neer glenoid.

Planning for the future – how to reduce revision rates

The best chance of a successful arthroplasty occurs at the first operation. It is the surgeon's responsibility to ensure that every primary operation carried out in his or her unit is completed as technically perfectly as possible. This applies particularly to hemiarthroplasties for acute trauma (four-part fractures and fracture dislocations), which, in the author's experience are associated with the highest failure rates. It will take another 5 years to discover if the porous coated glenoid component used to promote bone ingrowth will be more successful than the traditionally cemented glenoid component. Although the modular designs will allow easier revision surgery in the future, their use introduces further potential complications and the author has personal experience of the separation of one humeral head from a modular stem and three glenoid liners from uncemented glenoid bases. Some of the modular components may be associated with metal-to-metal contact after only a modest amount of wear has taken place, thus exposing the patient to excessive wear particles with their associated complications.

The additional problem of a large number of designs of implant, with each design being used on a relatively small number of patients, is also of concern and in the future the auditing of the outcome (as appreciated by the patients) will become increasingly important. It is hoped that manufacturers and surgeons may learn from their past mistakes in designing and inserting joint replacements, but only time – and appropriate follow-up studies – will verify if true progress is being made.

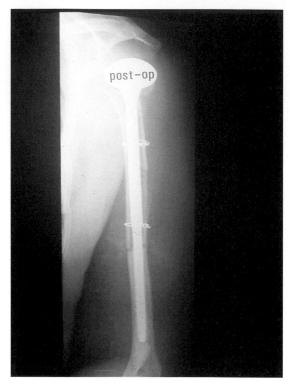

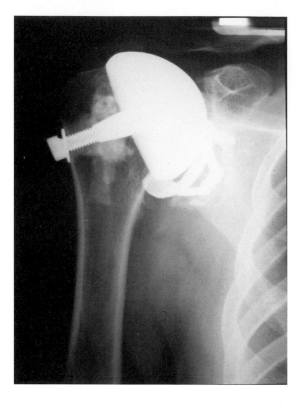

Figure 7.26 Loosening of the glenoid after 2 years; there was severe pain on using the arm.

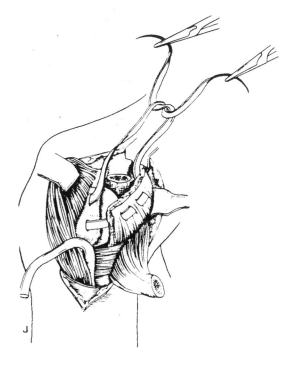

Figure 7.27 Postoperative position of revised shoulder arthroplasty in another patient using an allograft and biomodular components.

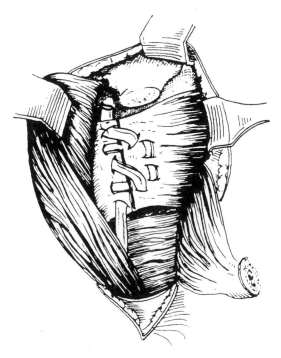

Figure 7.28 (a) and (b) Reconstruction of the tuberosities using Dacron tape.

References

Cofield RH and Edgerton BC (1990) Total shoulder arthroplasty: complications and revision surgery (Chapter 56). *Instructional Course Lectures, AAOS* **39** 449–462.

Dines DM, Warren RF, Altchek DW and Moeckel B (1993) Post-traumatic changes of the proximal humerus: malunion, nonunion and osteonecrosis. Treatment with modular hemiarthroplasty or total shoulder arthroplasty. *Journal of Shoulder and Elbow Surgery Hirst P and Wallace WA (1987) Poor results of Neer shoulder replacement in rheumatoid arthritis. In The Shoulder (N Takagishi, ed.), pp. 362–366. Tokyo: Professional Postgraduate Services.*

McCoy SR, Warren RF, Bade HA, Ranawat CS and Inglis AE (1989) Total shoulder arthroplasty in rheumatoid arthritis. *Journal of Arthroplasty* **4** 105–113.

Neer CS II, Watson KC and Stanton FJ (1982) Recent experience in total shoulder replacement *Journal of Bone and Joint Surgery* **64A** 319–337.

Redfern TR, Wallace WA and Beddow FH (1989) Clavicular osteotomy in shoulder arthroplasty. *International Orthopaedics* **13** 61–63.

Thomas BJ, Amstutz HC and Cracchiolo A (1991) Shoulder arthroplasty for rheumatoid arthritis. *Clinical Orthopaedics* **265** 125–128.

Vahvanen V, Hamalairen M, Paavolainen P (1989) The Neer II replacement for rheumatoid arthritis of the shoulder. *International Orthopedics* **13** 57–60.

Wallace WA (1990) The Nottingham Dacron hood reinforcement for unconstrained shoulder replacement. In. *Surgery of the Shoulder* (M. Post, BF Morrey and RJ Hawkins, eds), pp. 277–281. St Louis: Mosby–Year Book.

Wallace WA (1991) The shoulder. In *Atlas of Surgical Exposures* (CL Colton and AJ Hall, eds), pp. 134–146. Oxford: Butterworth–Heinemann.

Wallace WA, Schippinger G and Neumann L (1993) Reinforcement of the rotator cuff with the 'Nottingham (Terylene) hood'. Presented to the *7th Congress of the European Society for Surgery of the Shoulder and Elbow* (Aarhus, June 1993).

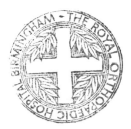

8

History of elbow arthroplasty

Peter G. Lunn and W. Angus Wallace

The elbow joint has long been acknowledged as playing an important role in the transmission of power to the upper limb. Phrases such as 'power to the elbow' and 'elbow grease' reflect the strength and rigidity required of the elbow, which perhaps was not fully recognized in the early days of the development of artificial elbow replacements. The complaint of the average rheumatoid patient with involvement of the elbow is primarily that of pain. Weakness is not usually mentioned because the progression of the disease is so gradual that the patient does not notice the slow but significant deterioration in strength. Nevertheless, the main functions of the elbow are to position the hand for normal everyday function and to stabilize the arm in order to allow power to be transmitted through the upper limb for load-bearing in tasks such as pushing up to get out of a chair.

Few reports of surgical treatment of the elbow are to be found in historical texts. The first excision arthroplasty of the elbow was probably performed in the sixteenth century as a remedy for intractable infection. Presumably the only alternative treatment at that time was amputation and there would be a high mortality associated with such a major surgical intervention. In relation to the ankle it had been reported by John Woodall that 'not more than four out of twenty lived till they had healed' after amputation of the foot at the ankle (Haeger, 1989). Syme in Edinburgh in 1831 wrote a *Treatise on the Excision of Diseased Joints*, in which he reported that the original idea of excision arthroplasty had come

from Mr Park of Liverpool. He reported a series of 14 patients treated with excision arthroplasty of the elbow, which he had started in 1828. Although two patients died and one required subsequent amputation, 11 had an acceptable outcome – much better results than he had experienced with primary amputation of the arm. Later, in 1878, Ollier in France published his extensive report on elbow arthrosis. He also wrote on the use of resection arthroplasty for patients who had suffered an ankylosis of the elbow in order to restore a functional range of movement. His paper not only indicated the limitation of resection arthroplasty but also demonstrated that patients with a stiff elbow often have a significant functional limitation and are generally keen to undergo any form of treatment in an attempt to restore movement.

The surgical treatments for arthritic pain in the elbow that have been developed over the years have concentrated on ways of removing what has appeared to be the source of the pain in an arthritic elbow – namely the deformed and eroded joint surfaces. These methods have included simple or radical excision arthroplasty, interposition arthroplasty (aimed at preventing contact between the joint surfaces) and the various types of prosthetic replacement of the joint. Three other treatments must also be considered: osteopathy, intra-articular steroid injections and synovectomy. The osteopath or bone-setter held a respected position as a reliever of pain: a simple manipulation for patients with elbow pain commonly produced dramatic pain relief. Steroid injection and synovectomy are both based on the hypothesis that the inflamed synovium is the origin of much of the pain and is also responsible for many of the changes in the joint which result in progressive destruction of the articular surfaces. Certainly in rheumatoid arthritis and some of the other inflammatory arthropathies dramatic and lasting relief has been obtained from both intra-articular steroids and from synovectomy; some of the implications of this will be discussed later.

Excision arthroplasty

In the nineteenth century the main indication for surgical treatment of the elbow was infection. Surgery was required either early, when incision and drainage of the pus was a life-saving procedure, or late, for the resulting painful destroyed joint or the ankylosed joint with poor function. Syme in 1837 (p. 212) stated that after septic arthritis: 'The elbow and shoulder joints while their structure and situation are most favourable for excision, hold out the greatest inducements to effect their removal without performing amputation.'

In the late situation excision arthroplasty seemed a reasonable method of treatment and it did have some measure of success but a number of problems were found to arise from simple excision of the joint. Excision arthroplasty of the hip had become a moderately successful procedure but in the elbow difficulty was found in preventing bony union between the bone ends of the humerus proximally and the ulna distally. Also, the relief of pain and the recovery of movements were variable and in some cases very poor. The elbow, like the knee, is a modified hinge joint and stability in one plane is important for useful function. In some of the more radical techniques, which involved the excision of a large amount of bone, a major instability problem frequently occurred (Figure 8.1) and occasionally required the use of a cumbersome external splint (Kirkaldy-Willis, 1948). A modern hinged orthosis is shown in Figure 8.2, but even today the provision of a splint which is acceptable and useful remains almost impossible.

As a result of poor pain relief, a limited range of movement and the risk of bony union across

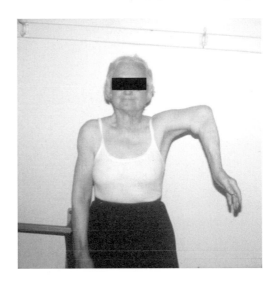

Figure 8.1 Major instability of the elbow may occur with resection arthroplasty, as shown here.

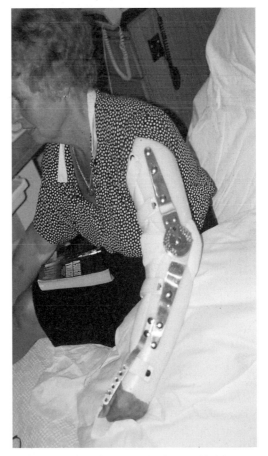

Figure 8.2 A modern hinged orthosis, moulded from polyethylene. This is still cumbersome and of limited value.

the excision arthroplasty site, the concept of an interposition arthroplasty developed.

Interposition arthroplasty

The search for a more predictable result from excision arthroplasty led surgeons in the late nineteenth century to try various materials interposed between the bone ends. These materials ranged from natural substances such as wood, gold, silver, tin and other metals, to synthetic sheets which included rubber and even animal tissues such as the lining of a pig's bladder. Later refinements, particularly the use of autologous fascia lata as the interposition membrane, led to an increase in the popularity of this technique in the first half of the twentieth century (MacAusland, 1921, 1948), with some remarkably successful results.

In Scandinavian countries, in particular, interposition arthroplasty has continued to be used in rheumatoid patients up to recent times and some of the best recorded results for any type of elbow arthroplasty have come from Finland using this technique (Laine and Vainio, 1969). Although Vainio and his colleagues have shown good results in terms of pain relief and patient satisfaction, other workers have shown unacceptable results in 20–50% of patients (Knight and van Zandt, 1952; Dee, 1969).

Arthrodesis of the elbow

From the early days of orthopaedic surgery, arthrodesis has always been the salvage procedure which the surgeon has felt can be resorted to if all else fails. A successful surgical fusion will result in stability of the joint and relief of the pain that previously occurred with movement. In cases of joint infection it has often been the treatment of choice. However, the elbow is not a good joint for arthrodesis because not only is reliable bony fusion difficult to achieve but, even if successful, the functional result is generally poor. Fusion of the elbow is difficult for two main reasons: firstly, the elbow is a difficult joint to immobilize effectively because of the long lever-arms of both the humerus and the forearm; secondly, there are usually only small areas for bony contact once the joint surfaces have been removed. Few series of elbow arthrodeses have been reported

in the literature but the paper by Koch and Lipscomb in 1967 illustrates the difficulty of this procedure: of the 17 cases in which an elbow arthrodesis was attempted, successful fusion was achieved in only eight patients (Koch and Lipscomb, 1967). It is possible that improvements in the techniques used for internal fixation, particularly the use of AO (Arbeitsgemeinschaft für Osteosynthesefragen) compression plate fixation, may be more successful at achieving fusion, but the indications for an arthrodesis are now very limited in our present-day practice. This is partly because our patients in the 1990s have a greater expectation for the outcome of treatment and partly because other surgical treatments are becoming available, but in addition the spectrum of disease has altered significantly in the last 50 years: the incidence of joint infection has reduced considerably and tuberculosis, which used to be a common cause of bone and joint infection, is now rarely seen. In some parts of the world, particularly in less developed countries, this may not be the case and arthrodesis can still be a valuable operation in such a situation. However, it is helpful to heed the words of MacAusland (1921) who stated: 'In the elbow, on the other hand, no position of ankylosis is favourable to function and any position is ungainly.'

Osteotomy for elbow pain

Osteotomy around the elbow has never been popular for relieving pain and retaining motion in arthritic conditions. It may be that the long lever-arm effect causes delayed or non-union of the osteotomy, or that surgery around the elbow is often associated with permanent joint stiffness, which would almost certainly jeopardize the functional result. The results of osteotomy for other joints in rheumatoid arthritis are variable and some authorities feel that osteotomy is often of such limited value generally that it should be abandoned for the management of the rheumatoid patient.

Synovectomy for the painful rheumatoid elbow

Synovectomy is a technique that has some strong advocates and it has enjoyed some considerable success in the past. Again, the Scandinavians have had the greatest experience and success with synovectomy – much more than other surgeons in Europe or in North America. Vainio reported a series of 92 patients who had undergone elbow synovectomy, of whom 75% achieved a satisfactory result in terms of pain relief (Laine and Vainio, 1969). Savill in 1971, from Edinburgh, reported a series of 14 patients of whom 11 obtained 'complete relief of pain'. These patients were usually selected at a very early stage of the disease process before there was any significant evidence of radiological change as Savill had found the results much less satisfactory once erosions were present on X-ray. The largest published series on elbow synovectomy, with radial head excision, is that by Porter, Richardson and Vainio (1974) who found that of 154 elbows reviewed, 70% of patients were pleased but the radiographic outcome was only 'satisfactory' in 54% of cases. They commented that synovectomy gave only short-lived good results when carried out for advanced rheumatoid disease of the elbow.

Radial head excision

Excision of the radial head has been carried out for many years, with satisfactory results in a large proportion of patients. It is mainly indicated for localized radiocapitellar arthritis, for example after a malunited radial head fracture. This operation has also been used in rheumatoid arthritis, really as a part of 'debridement' procedure in which the radial head is removed, partly because of the erosive changes on the articular surface but also in order to gain access to the inside of the elbow to carry out as radical a synovectomy as possible. No implant was inserted and a fibrous pseudarthrosis was allowed to develop.

Subsequently some surgeons developed the view that by carrying out an excision arthroplasty at the elbow, problems at the wrist joint might occur as a result of the long-term radial shortening and secondary subluxation at the distal radioulnar joint. Swanson developed a silicone radial head implant in the hope that this would prevent deformity occurring both at the elbow and at the wrist. He started using this technique in 1967 (Swanson and Herndon, 1982) and the early results were encouraging,

both in terms of pain relief and range of movement in the elbow and forearm. Later reports from other centres showed that the longer-term results were less satisfactory and there was cause for concern with regard to fragmentation of the silicone implant. The severe giant-cell reaction which has been associated with some cases of silicone fragmentation in the region of the wrist has not been seen to the same extent in the elbow.

It is partly because of the doubts raised about the longevity of silicone in this situation that more long-lasting designs of radial head implant have been developed. Miller in Glasgow and Amis in London have developed a vitallium implant which is currently undergoing clinical trials (Amis and Miller, 1984). At the present time it is not possible to say whether or not radial head implants should be used in some or all patients, nor indeed whether there is a suitable implant which can stand the test of time.

Development of prosthetic elbow joints

The development and introduction of elbow arthroplasty will now be reviewed and the present progress and potential future developments will be explored. It is interesting to reflect that, in some respects, elbow arthroplasty appeared on the orthopaedic scene a little too early and if it had developed some 10 years later one wonders whether some of the lessons learnt from lower limb arthroplasties would have influenced the designers of the earlier elbow prostheses. Sadly, this 'overview' of the history of elbow arthroplasty will demonstrate that many of the lessons which have now been learned in the lower limb, particularly from knee arthroplasty, have been relearned in the elbow. Common mistakes were repeated and only now, as a better understanding of the underlying biomechanics of the elbow joint has been acquired, has it been possible to develop elbow prostheses with a more predictable outcome in both the short and long term.

Hemiarthroplasty

Street and Stevens in 1974 reported on their experience using a metallic hemiarthroplasty to resurface the distal end of the humerus. This had only a limited application because it required good bone stock of the distal humerus and this is frequently not present, particularly in rheumatoid patients. It was perhaps more applicable to post-traumatic osteoarthritic cases. Unfortunately, like hemiarthroplasty of other joints, the results proved unpredictable and this prosthesis has largely been superseded by total elbow arthroplasty.

Total elbow arthroplasty

The development of total arthroplasty has progressed along a steep learning curve strongly influenced by an increasing awareness of the biomechanics of the elbow joint and also the physical characteristics of the interface between the bone, the implant and, when used, the cement.

Rigid hinges

There are reports of some hinged elbow implants implanted into patients on a 'one off' basis from as long ago as 1942 (Knight and van Zandt, 1952), but it was not until the 1970s that development of elbow arthroplasties really caught the interest of the orthopaedic world.

In Britain, it was Dee (1969) who led the way with a hinged elbow arthroplasty, with early work also taking place at the Royal National Orthopaedic Hospital in London (Scales, Lettin and Bayley, 1977) (Figure 8.3), while Coonrad in the USA and Gschwend in Europe (Gschwend, Scheier and Bahler, 1977) also developed rigid hinged implants. The early results in some cases were dramatic in terms of pain relief, range of movement and return of function.

An important milestone in the development of these prostheses came in 1973 when Souter published the results of hinged arthroplasties carried out in 20 rheumatoid patients over the previous 3 years (Souter, 1973). In his conclusions he recognized that the short-term results were good but he advised caution about the long-term results because of the early signs of loosening with a number of these prostheses. As these early fears were realized over the next few years the design of elbow prostheses has altered significantly.

Semiconstrained linked hinges

In the 1970s, Swanson experimented with a

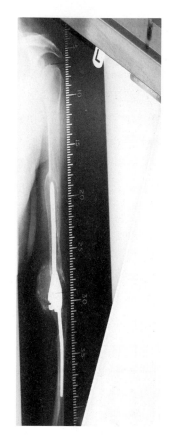

Figure 8.3 Stanmore total elbow replacement with signs of gross loosening.

silicone flexible hinge (Swanson and Herndon, 1982) but this was not sufficiently strong and it fragmented with use. Latterly, Pritchard (1977), in particular, developed a floppy linked hinge arthroplasty which had some built-in flexibility so that although it did confer some stability it was anticipated that it would be less likely to loosen because there would be reduced stresses on the fixation compared with the earlier rigid hinges. Neither of these prostheses has become popular.

Semiconstrained unlinked prostheses

The bioengineers have now concluded that the reason for failure of the rigid hinges was that the fixation could not withstand the very large forces transmitted across the elbow joint and thus to the implant. There was no way of improving the fixation of the constrained implants and so the only other way of dealing with the problem was to design the prosthesis in

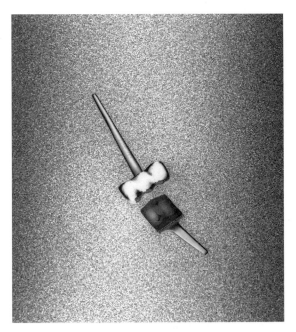

Figure 8.4 Capitello-Condylar™ total elbow replacement. (™ – Trade-mark of Johnson & Johnson Professional. Photograph supplied courtesy of Johnson & Johnson Professional – Orthopaedic division.)

such a way as to reduce the stresses acting across it; hence the unlinked prostheses which will allow the soft tissues (ligaments and capsule) to absorb a large proportion of the forces, thereby reducing the stresses on the bone–cement interface.

The early designs of unlinked prostheses were minimally constrained and required minimal bone resection. They were therefore inherently much more satisfactory for subsequent salvage procedures than hinged arthroplasties which often required a large amount of bone resection and were associated with a considerable amount of bone resorption when they loosened.

As experience with unconstrained prostheses increased, it became clear that the lack of constraint of these prostheses rendered them more vulnerable to instability, and the design of some, particularly those associated with minimal bone resection, did not allow a sufficiently large prosthesis-to-bone contact area for adequate fixation of the components. Some of these earlier prostheses such as the ICHL (Roper et al, 1986), the Lowe–Miller (Lowe et al, 1984) and the Cavendish were subsequently modified in order to give better fixation.

Ewald in Boston, USA, developed an unconstrained elbow arthroplasty with a long humeral stem fixation and a polyethylene ulnar component and with less inherent constraint in the prosthesis. This was first inserted in 1974 but has been modified since (Figure 8.4) and his results (Ewald et al, 1980) have been very satisfactory in rheumatoid patients, although there were early problems with dislocation of the prosthesis. Additional results from the use of this design by other surgeons have been very encouraging and currently the Ewald elbow has been used more frequently than any other.

Souter, in Edinburgh, in conjunction with the Bioengineering Department at the University of Strathclyde, developed a similar, semiconstrained, unlinked arthroplasty with a short humeral stem but fashioned in such a way as to give as secure rotational fixation in bone as possible (Figure 8.5). This was first used in 1977, with the only major modification being the introduction of a long-stemmed humeral revision component in 1988. The medium-term results have been encouraging, but again only in rheumatoid patients.

Both these surgeons have now built up a very large experience of elbow arthroplasty and both are now reporting series of more than 100 patients over more than 5 years follow-up, with good results. It appears that the fixation of these prostheses is very much more secure and, as a result of improved surgical technique, the stability after insertion is now satisfactory.

The third elbow prosthesis gaining in popularity is the Kudo prosthesis, developed in Japan. In fact these are a range of prostheses, starting in 1972 with the Type 1 – a surface replacement. The design was modified in 1975 to a more physiological shape with an intramedullary stem on the ulnar component – the Type 2. In 1983 the design was very significantly further modified to the Type 3 by the addition of intramedullary stems to both components. In 1985 the Type 2 prosthesis was discontinued, and in 1988 the Type 3 was modified with the addition of titanium alloy stems with porous coating – the Type 4 (Figure 8.6). Although Kudo and Iwano have reported the long-term results of the 'Kudo elbow' (Kudo and Iwano, 1990), the results refer to prostheses no longer in use; we await the outcome from the Type 4 over the next 10 years.

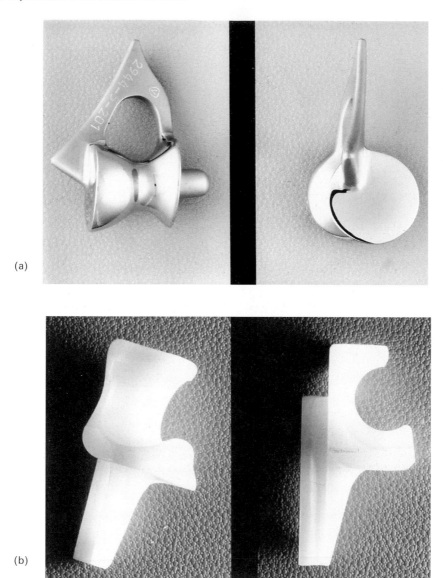

Figure 8.5 (a) and (b) Souter–Strathclyde total elbow replacement.

The future of elbow arthroplasty

At the present time it has become clear that there is a definite need for an effective elbow arthroplasty for rheumatoid patients and it may well be that the present semiconstrained prostheses, with adequate fixation, will meet this need in a large number of patients. There are some, however, who need the extra stability afforded by a hinged prosthesis and it appears that some form of 'flexible' hinge is still required. There are also a number of elderly patients with primary osteoarthritis and young patients with post-traumatic arthritis who pose a major clinical problem. Surgeons who have occasionally tried arthroplasty for osteoarthritis have usually had major problems with component loosening as these patients expect to return to normal activities and the bone–cement interface does not stand up to normal everyday stresses. Perhaps the advent of bone ingrowth will improve fixation but this is as yet unproven and these osteoarthritic patients are currently not satisfactorily catered for.

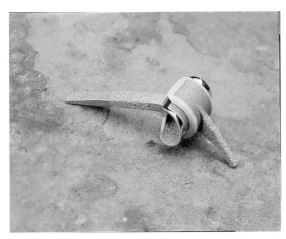

Figure 8.6 Kudo (Type 4) total elbow replacement. (Courtesy of Biomet Ltd.)

The future therefore holds much hope for restoring the 'power to the elbow' for the rheumatoid patient, but there needs to be further development before we can offer similar hope of pain relief and power to the osteo-arthritic patients in whom the mechanical demands from the arthroplasty are often much greater than in the rheumatoid patient.

References

Amis AA and Miller JH (1984) Design, development, and clinical trial of a modular elbow replacement incorporating cement-free fixation. *Engineering in Medicine* **13** 175–179.

Dee R (1969) Elbow arthroplasty. *Proceedings of the Royal Society of Medicine* **62** 1031–1035.

Ewald FC, Scheinberg RD, Poss R, Thomas WH, Scott RD and Sledge CB (1980) Capitello-condylar total elbow arthroplasty: two to five year follow-up in rheumatoid arthritis. *Journal of Bone and Joint Surgery* **62A** 1259–1263.

Gschwend N, Scheier H and Bahler A (1977) GSB elbow-, wrist-, and PIP joints, In *Joint Replacement in the Upper Limb*, pp. 107–116. London: Institution of Mechanical Engineers.

Haeger K (1989) *The Illustrated History of Surgery*, p. 219. London: Harold Starke.

Kirkaldy-Willis WH (1948) Excision of the elbow joint. *Lancet* **i** 53–57.

Knight RA and van Zandt IL (1952) Arthroplasty of the elbow – an end result study. *Journal of Bone and Joint Surgery* **36A** 610–618.

Koch M and Lipscomb PR (1967) Arthrodesis of the elbow. *Clinical Orthopaedics* **50** 151–157.

Kudo H and Iwano K (1990) Total elbow arthroplasty with a non-constrained surface-replacement prosthesis in patients who have rheumatoid arthritis. *Journal of Bone and Joint Surgery* **72A** 355–362.

Laine V and Vainio K (1969) Synovectomy of the elbow. In *Early Synovectomy in Rheumatoid Arthritis* (W Hijmans, WD Paul and H Herschel, eds), pp. 117–118. Amsterdam: Excerpta Medica.

Lowe LW, Miller AJ, Allum RL and Higginson DW (1984) The development of an unconstrained elbow arthroplasty – a clinical review. *Journal of Bone and Joint Surgery* **66B** 243–247.

MacAusland WR (1921) Mobilisation of the elbow by free fascia transplantation. *Surgery, Gynecology and Obstetrics* **33** 223–245.

MacAusland WR (1948) Arthroplasty of the elbow. *New England Journal of Medicine* **236** 97–99.

Ollier L (1878) De la resection du coude dans les cas d'ankylose. *Revue de Médicine et de Chirurgie* **6**.

Porter BB, Richardson C and Vainio K (1974) Rheumatoid arthritis of the elbow, the results of synovectomy. *Journal of Bone and Joint Surgery* **56B** 427–437.

Pritchard RW (1977) Flexible elbow replacement. In *Joint Replacement in the Upper Limb*, pp. 63–68. London: Institution of Mechanical Engineers.

Roper BA, Tuke M, O'Riordan SM and Bulstrode CJ (1986) A new unconstrained elbow. A prospective review of 60 replacements. *Journal of Bone and Joint Surgery* **68B** 566–569.

Savill DL (1971) Synovectomy and debridement of the rheumatoid elbow. Paper presented to the ABC Travelling Fellows, Princess Margaret Rose Hospital.

Scales JT, Lettin AWF and Bayley I (1977) The evolution of the Stanmore hinged total elbow replacement 1967–1976. In *Joint Replacement in the Upper Limb*, pp. 53–62. London: Institution of Mechanical Engineers.

Souter WA (1973) Arthroplasty of the elbow – with particular reference to metallic hinge arthroplasty in rheumatoid patients. *Orthopedic Clinics of North America* **4** 395–413.

Street DM and Stevens PS (1974) A humeral replacement prosthesis for the elbow. *Journal of Bone and Joint Surgery* **56A** 1147–1158.

Swanson AB and Herndon JH (1982) Surgery of arthritis. In *The Elbow* (TG Wadsworth, ed.), pp. 303–345. Edinburgh: Churchill Livingstone.

Syme J (1831) *Treatise on the Excision of Diseased Joints*. Edinburgh: published by Longmans predecessor.

Syme J (1837) *The Principles of Surgery*, pp. 199, 212. Edinburgh: Carfrae and Son, Maclachlan and Stewart.

9

Biomechanics of the elbow

Andrew A. Amis

The major function of the upper limb is to move and support the hand in the space around the body during all activities. The mobility of the shoulder joint allows a wide arc for the basic limb direction, but it is the elbow which must flex and extend through large ranges of motion to control the distance of the hand from the body, such as in reaching for objects or bringing food to the mouth. The function of the elbow is complicated by the need to accommodate forearm rotation, the hand being pronated to pick up an object and supinated to receive an object or to bring it to the mouth.

The length of lever represented by the forearm and hand means that the external forces acting on the hand in many activities are remote from the axis of movement of the elbow, while the muscles which move and stabilize the joint can only pass close to its axis. The resulting short lever arms of the muscles mean that the muscle tensions must be very much higher than the external loads, and this leads to correspondingly large loads being imposed on the joint by the muscles. Thus, although the skeleton of the upper limb is much less massive than in the legs, the stresses applied to the bones and joints are similar; the loads are transmitted by smaller areas of articular cartilage and the bones have thinner cortices. The result is that joint replacement surgery, for example, will be more difficult than in the lower limb because the great mobility of the elbow causes loosening forces to attack the fixation of

a small implant from a wide range of directions.

A mobile joint which has large forces imposed on it from different directions is obviously in need of adequate stabilization. Electromyographic studies, discussed below, have shown that the elbow is routinely stabilized by antagonistic muscle contractions that pack the joint surfaces together. However, this mechanism still relies on a system of ligaments and capsular structures to stabilize the joint in many activities.

Disruption of the co-ordinated functions of the elbow joint surfaces, muscles and ligaments leads to severe impairment of upper limb function, whether arising from trauma or disease, particularly because of the elbow's propensity to stiffen in response to any insult. Although elbow problems affect the activities of daily life in the majority of rheumatoid patients (Amis et al, 1982), the upper limb has attracted much less research attention than the lower limb. Early designs of elbow joint prostheses, for example, were designed and in use before the joint forces had been analysed in depth. It is intended that the biomechanical data presented below will provide some informed guidelines for surgeons faced with reconstituting the elbow. The chapter will start with a detailed description of the articular geometry, which is essential if the joint motions are to be understood. The muscle actions causing joint motion and then the forces which they impose on the joint will be described, followed by an examination of the function of the forearm in transmitting forces such as arise in falls on to the outstretched hand.

Articular geometry and contact areas

The subtle shaping of the elbow joint surfaces has led to much debate regarding the motion of the forearm bones in relation to the humerus during flexion or rotation activities. The basic shapes of the bobbin-like trochlea beside the spherical capitellum are well known, but there have been various descriptions published which suggest a more complex behaviour than a simple hinge motion about a fixed axis during flexion.

Although Dempster (1955) and Burrough (1973) found that sagittal sections of the joint were close to circles, Fick (1911), Steindler (1964) and Ewald (1975) suggested that the capitellum was placed eccentrically to the trochlea when viewed laterally and had a spiral contour which moved the centre of rotation and caused a longitudinal shift of the radius relative to the ulna during flexion. Observing that the medial facet of the olecranon is exposed in extension, while the lateral facet is exposed in flexion (Figure 9.1a), Fick (1911) proposed that the trochlear shape incorporates a screw-thread effect which moves the ulna laterally in flexion. Similarly, Kapandji (1970) proposed that different axes within the trochlea were dominant in flexion and extension to cause the carrying angle variation, while Morrey and Chao (1976) noted a small ulnar rotation into supination during flexion.

The elbow articulation has also been reported to change with ageing, Goodfellow and Bullough (1967) noting degeneration and cartilage loss from the humero-radial articulation, followed by a wearing-in of the humeroulnar joint. Yamaguchi (1972) showed a sequence of trochlear notch degeneration from an entire cartilage covering to a two-part notch (distal and proximal articular parts) (Figure 9.1b).

The shapes of the bones and the congruence of the joints can be studied in detail by means of acrylic replicas made by pouring liquid bone cement into silicone rubber moulds of cadaveric bones. The accuracy of this replication was shown by Seedhom et al (1973). The replica joints can be embedded into a contrasting colour at different angles of flexion, then sliced for analysis. This method showed that the

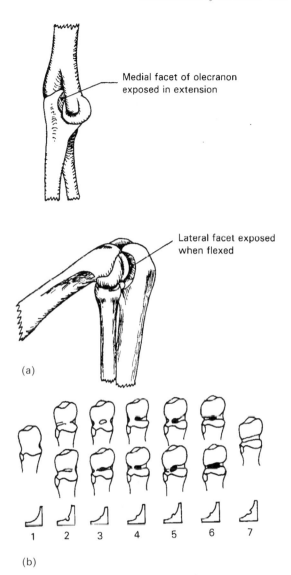

(a)

(b)

Figure 9.1 (a) Exposure of the medial facet of the olecranon in extension and the lateral facet in flexion. (b) Sequence of trochlear notch degeneration: 1 = none; 7 = complete separation of articular cartilage of notch into proximal and distal parts (Yamaguchi, 1992).

elbow had surfaces close to circles in the sagittal plane in young specimens, typically within 0.2 mm from a particular diameter (Amis, 1978). The deviation from a circle led to elliptical humeral sections which wedged between the coronoid and olecranon (Figure 9.2a). This geometry distorted in older specimens, as the trochlear notch cartilage separated into two facets (Figure 9.2b). Surprisingly, however, this obviously out-of-round geometry still allows the humeroulnar joint to move

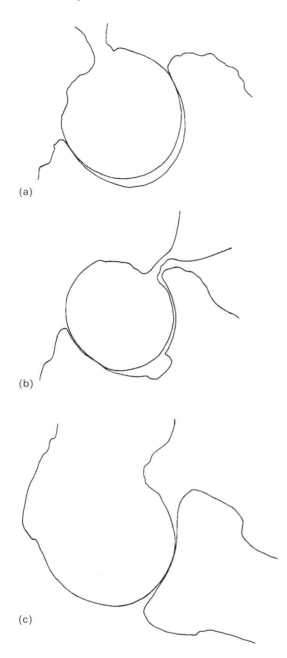

(a)

(b)

(c)

Figure 9.2 (a) The trochlea of the humerus is slightly elliptical, resulting in joint incongruity. (b) Incongruity is greater in older specimens, when the trochlear notch is separated into two parts. (c) A different form of incongruity of joint surfaces is seen in the humeroradial joint.

within ± 0.3 mm of a fixed axis during flexion. A typical humeroradial articulation is seen in Figure 9.2c, which shows an accurate hemisphere for the capitellum, blending to a larger radius posteriorly. The concave end face of the

radius is not congruent with the capitellum, and the resulting small central contact area will lead to high localized cartilage stresses in use. This explains the pathology noted by Goodfellow and Bullough (1967). This geometry will give uniaxial motion in flexion, apart from a shift in the centre of rotation as the radius approaches full extension.

Further analysis of the joint sections showed that the centres of the circular approximations to the sagittal sections all lay within 1.2 mm of a straight line, even in elderly joints. This means that the radius and ulna both effectively move around the same fixed axis during flexion–extension, and do not move relative to each other. This finding confirms that a single axis will give accurate joint motion in a prosthesis, which is as a consequence much easier to make, and these findings have been confirmed radiographically (London, 1981) and by dissection (Sorbie et al, 1986). The apparent eccentricity of the capitellum to the trochlea reported by Ewald (1975) is thus seen to be because a view perpendicular to the humerus is not along the articular axis, which is slanting. This was suggested by Potter in 1895 and confirmed by cadaveric measurement by Amis et al in 1977 and later radiographically by London in 1981. The axis bisects the angle between arm and forearm in full extension, causing the normal carrying angle variation described below.

Slicing across the width of the joint surfaces in planes parallel to the flexion axis shows that not only is the capitellum spherical, but so too are the two facets of the trochlea throughout most of their extent (Figure 9.3). This geometry is the only one which can maintain a large contact area if the ulna is abducted or adducted from its mean position of resting on the two facets. Posteriorly, the lateral facet of the trochlea becomes concave and sweeps up on to the side of the olecranon fossa. In full extension, a small lateral facet of the olecranon, which is rarely recognized, wedges here to stabilize the ulna against varus angulation. Examination of Figure 9.3 shows that the lateral/medial gaping of the joint in flexion/extension is not due to sideways movement of the ulna but is a result of the end faces of the trochlea not being perpendicular to the flexion axis.

There have been several reports of elbow joint contact area studies. Dempster (1955) and Burrough (1973) reported a concentration on

FLEXED POSITION

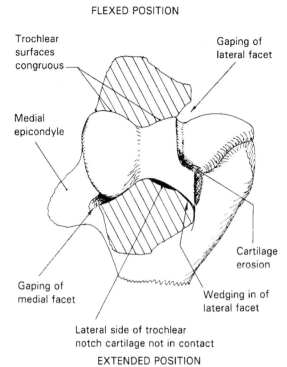

Figure 9.3 The shape of the trochlea with its medial and lateral facets related to the olecranon, shown sectioned in flexion and extension.

the central ridge of the trochlear notch. Goodfellow and Bullough (1967) noted that the centre of the radial head always contacted the capitellum and that its triangular medial facet contacted the radial notch of the ulna during forearm rotation. The humero-ulnar joint contacted in two zones, extending across the width of the joint; this was also found by Walker (1977).

Of the above workers, only Walker applied a load (500 N) greater than hand pressure. The present author used the silicone rubber casting method of Seedhom and Tsubuku (1977), in which liquid rubber is squeezed out of the joint while it is loaded in a compression test machine. When set, the contact areas are revealed as holes in the rubber. Figure 9.4 shows typical humeroulnar results for a 50 N load for several angles of flexion. Increases in the loading to 1.5 kN caused the contact areas to increase until most of the articulation was in contact. Pronating the ulna, as allowed by slackness of the medial collateral ligament, caused the contact to roll on to one of the spherical facets of the trochlea. Measurement of the contact

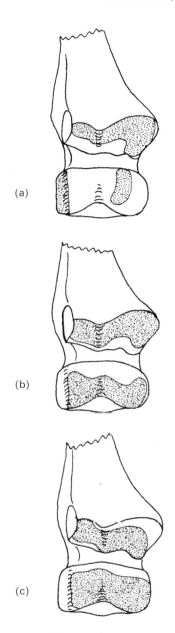

Figure 9.4 Typical humeroulnar contact areas with an applied joint force of 50 N.

areas showed that the humero-radial joint cartilage was subjected to much higher contact stresses than the trochlea in response to a given load, and the contact area remained at the centre of the end face of the radius.

The overall shape of the elbow joint was described by Street and Stevens (1974), as the basis for a humeral hemiarthroplasty prosthesis for the elbow, but direct measurements on cadaveric joints by the present author found

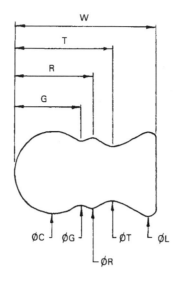

Dimension	Mean (% width)	Standard deviation	Correlation coefficient	Cadaver survey (% width)
T	66.2	2.7	0.92	66.5
R	48.1	2.4	0.90	46.5
G	38.4	2.6	0.82	-
ØC	53.9	4.4	0.70	51.1
ØG	45.1	4.3	0.59	-
ØR	50.7	3.8	0.73	48.9
ØT	40.5	4.1	0.56	39.4
ØL	63.2	6.3	0.59	62.2

Figure 9.5 Direct measurement of the dimensions of the trochlea taken from 100 radiographs, plus cadaver measurements normalized as % of W.

some differences. A review of 100 radiographs (Amis et al, 1977) gave results matching the direct measurements (Figure 9.5), showing that the articular surfaces have a constant shape which only varies in scale from one elbow to another. This review showed that male elbows were significantly larger than female. It was not possible to extend this analysis to the bone shafts adjacent to the joint, the angulations and sizes of the bones depending on factors such as the strength and build of individuals. For the radius, the head had a mean thickness of 49% of its diameter, but the neck diameter varied so

much for a given head size that one neck could fit within the medulla of another. Similarly, the proximal shaft of the ulna varied from 6 to 23° from the sagittal plane, with a mean of 14°. These variable factors make it difficult to design implant fixation stems which will be a good fit in all elbows.

Elbow movements

In normal activities, elbow movements are but one component of the complex inter-relationships that comprise the fluent function of the upper limb: flexion–extension and pronation–supination are mixed together in varying degrees. Analysis of such 'normal' activity remains largely in the realm of laboratory-based research, using methods such as multi-camera cine photography (Nicol, 1977) or complex multiaxis goniometers (Chao et al, 1980).

Flexion–extension motion

This movement is generally regarded as a 'hinge' motion centred in the distal humeral articulation, with flexion commencing from the extended anatomical position of the upper limb. There has been considerable debate as to the exact nature of this movement within the elbow articulations, often complicated by authors seeking simultaneously to explain the concurrent variations of the carrying angle. This debate has little relevance to clinical measurements of elbow motion, as the axis does not move significantly, but it is important if a precise knowledge is needed, such as when designing a prosthesis. The literature falls into two groups: those who found a fixed centre of rotation (Potter, 1895; Hultkrantz, 1897; Youm et al, 1979; London, 1981); and those who found moving instantaneous centres (Fischer, 1907; Dempster, 1955; Ewald, 1975; Morrey and Chao, 1976). Of these, only Dempster (1955) found a significant movement (12.5 mm). Amis (1978) found that the axis of movement was always within a radius of 0.3 mm at the centre of the trochlea, which is not surprising in view of the articular surfaces having approximately circular sections, as noted above. It may be concluded that for all practical purposes the forearm flexes in a circular arc about a single fixed axis passing through the centres of both capitellum and trochlea. It is probable that much of the reported deviation from uniaxial motion has arisen from inaccuracies in the experimental work.

The accepted method for describing forearm flexion is that of Cave and Roberts (1936), which was adopted by a Combined Meeting of the Orthopaedic Associations of the English-speaking World (American Academy of Orthopedic Surgeons, 1966). This system defines the fully extended elbow as 0° flexion, with a mean range of 142°, the latter figure being a mean of published measurements of adult males (Amis and Miller, 1982). Prior to 1966, most American publications used Clark's system (1920), which quoted the angle between limb segments, so that the 'elbow angle' had full extension at 180° and full flexion at 38°.

Some people can extend the elbow beyond the straight line, into hyperextension, a phenomenon more common in females. Fick (1911) found that females extended an average of 5° more than males and Sinelnikoff and Grigoro-witsch (1931) found an 8° difference. Hyperextension has been linked to the presence of a supratrochlear foramen (Zimmer, 1968), an aperture linking the coronoid and olecranon fossae, thus delaying humero-ulnar impingement.

Since active flexion is limited by apposition of the tensed flexor muscles against the forearm, passive motion would be expected to be greater, the relaxed muscles then allowing motion to be limited by bone to bone contact: Glanville and Kreezer (1937) found an increase of 5° flexion. Similarly, slim subjects have an average of 10° greater active flexion than muscular or obese subjects (Sinelnikoff and Grigorowitsch, 1931; Barter, Emanuel and Truett, 1957; Hertzberg, 1972). The range of motion decreases significantly with age: children in the first decade have an average hyperextension of 6° (West, 1945; Silverman et al, 1975), while the onset of middle age is associated with flexion decreasing by 5° (Boone and Azen, 1979).

Forearm rotation

Forearm rotation is normally described by splitting the movement into arcs of pronation and supination from a neutral position. This is usually defined, and positioned in the clinic, as the hand being in a sagittal plane, palm medially, with the elbow flexed 90° and the arm

alongside the body. This posture aims to eliminate humeral motion from measurements of forearm rotation. Other postures can give different results, partly because humeral rotation may occur, partly because of different muscle tensions, such as in the biceps crossing both the shoulder and the elbow. Thus Salter and Darcus (1953) showed that, although the hand can rotate further with the elbow extended, there is then less rotation in the forearm itself.

The classical anatomical description of forearm rotation is that the radius swings around the stationary ulna, like the handle on a bucket (Patrick, 1946). The radius is constrained to have such a motion relative to the ulna by the annular ligament surrounding the radial head and by the triangular fibrocartilage tethering the distal radius to the ulnar head. This description would be complete if the ulna were to remain stationary during forearm rotation but this, of course, implies that the hand would swing about an axis coincident with the little finger. Normal forearm rotation, however, takes place about an axis at the centre of the wrist, as demonstrated by Taylor and Blaschke (1948) and Capener (1956), so there must also be ulnar motion. The nature (and even existence) of this motion is still not accepted generally, some authors feeling that the lateral ulnar movements arise at the humero-ulnar joint, while others suggest that they arise from humeral rotations. This disagreement is surprising in view of the elegant experiments on cadavers by Heiberg (1884) and Dwight (1884), supplemented by experiments in vivo by Ray, Johnson and Jameson (1951). Heiberg immobilized the humerus, disarticulated the hand, and inserted paintbrushes into the ends of the radius and ulna. The wrist was rotated within a ring and arcs of radial and ulnar motion were painted, thus proving humeroulnar motion in the cadaver. Dwight added detail by demonstrating that the arcuate ulnar motion was circumduction – transverse pins through the ulna showed that the motion did not include rotation. Thus, for forearm rotations away from the neutral position, pronation involves ulnar abduction and flexion, while supination involves adduction and flexion (Figure 9.6). Ray, Johnson and Jameson (1951) proved that this lateral angular motion occurs at the elbow in living subjects by pinning the epicondyles to a fixed frame, constraining motion to certain

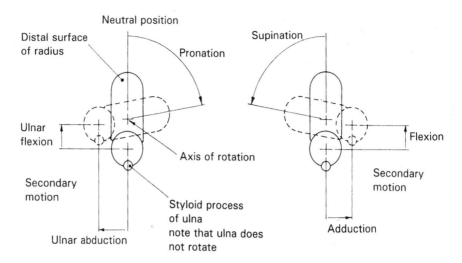

Figure 9.6 When the forearm rotates, pronation involves ulnar abduction and flexion, while supination involves ulnar adduction and flexion.

axes by tension on a Chinese finger-basket and then using double-exposed radiographs at the limits of rotation. They showed a mean arc of 9° of lateral ulnar motion, which implies that the elbow collateral ligaments must be slightly slack.

The amplitude of forearm rotation is extremely variable, and it is generally recognized that a normal contralateral limb should be used as a reference. Clinical measurements are best done with a hand-held pendulum goniometer (Patrick 1946) but, although convenient, readings obtained can be augmented by 'trick' movements within the hand. A wrist cuff goniometer measures only the forearm rotation and is more suitable for clinical research. Darcus and Salter (1953) found a mean difference of 27° rotation between hand and wrist goniometers; they also noted that the hand was supinated an average of 11° from the forearm. A review of earlier literature carried out by Amis and Miller (1982) found mean ranges of pronation/supination of 76°/80° at the wrist, and 77°/106° at the hand. Glanville and Kreezer (1937) found that passive rotation of the hand caused a mean increase of 30° rotation. Female subjects had an average of 8° more forearm rotation than males in the study of Salter and Darcus (1953). The effect of age was reported by Boone and Azen (1979), who found that under-fives had more pronation and supination than young adults, while over-forties had a significant decrease in supination.

Carrying angle

The carrying angle causes the forearm to deviate laterally from the arm when the elbow is extended, giving a characteristic shape that can be deformed by malunion of supracondylar fractures (Smith, 1960). Despite the apparent simplicity of this angulation there is much confusion in the literature on how to define it, or measure it, or how it varies with flexion, or what is normal. This has arisen largely from the publication of many bizarre definitions linked to the position of the ulna, the medial outline of the soft tissues, etc., rather than keeping to what is seen by both patient and clinician: 'the deviation of the perceived centreline of the supinated forearm from the sagittal plane containing the humeral axis' (Amis et al, 1977). This applies at any angle of flexion, but is only easily measured in the clinic at full extension, when it is largest. What is required is an angle of abduction of the forearm in the plane in which the forearm would move if the collateral ligaments allowed it, at any angle of flexion. These measurements have been made using the goniometer shown in Figure 9.7, which was fixed to the humerus of cadavers and allowed the wrist to slide laterally during flexion. A typical result (Figure 9.8) shows that laxity of the collateral ligaments allowed a range of abduction and adduction of the forearm, at any angle of flexion of approximately 9°. This confirmed the ulnar mobility

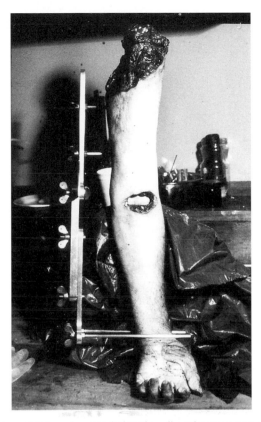

Figure 9.7 A goniometer designed to allow the measurement of the variation of the carrying angle in different degrees of elbow flexion.

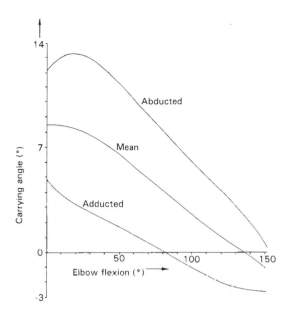

Figure 9.8 The results for the carrying angle (in the stressed abduction and stressed adduction positions) for one cadaver.

reported by Ray, Johnson and Jameson (1951) during forearm rotation. The mean motion corresponded closely to a sinusoidal reduction of the carrying angle during flexion, which occurred because the flexion axis bisected the angle between arm and forearm in full extension (Amis et al, 1977). This mechanism was originally proposed by Potter (1895) and means that the axis of an elbow prosthesis, for example, should be inclined perhaps 6° from a line perpendicular to the long axis of the humerus, when it will also be approximately 6° from a line perpendicular to the long axis of the forearm. London (1981) reported that the carrying angle remained constant with flexion, which was correct in relation to the tilted humeral flexion axis which he used as a constant datum, rather than the sagittal plane. A report by Morrey and Chao (1976), that the carrying angle varied linearly with flexion and that the forearm was in varus when fully flexed, should be treated with reserve because their

measurements ignored the lateral angular movements allowed by the collateral ligament laxity.

The mean carrying angle in extension was found to be 11° in adult males and 14° in adult females when published data were reviewed (Amis and Miller, 1982). Smith (1960) found that children had a smaller mean carrying angle of 5° for males and 6° for females, so only small inaccuracies in the reduction of supracondylar fractures will lead to 'gunstock' deformities.

Muscle actions

Muscle actions are normally studied by electromyography, in which electrical activity is monitored using wire electrodes embedded into individual muscles, or by surface electrodes taped to the skin (Basmajian, 1967). If this literature is to be used to provide data in analysis of joint forces, then the investigator must ensure that the results relate to strenuous situations. For example, Basmajian and Latif (1957) noted little biceps activity during flexion of a pronated forearm, whereas Pauly, Rushing and Scheving (1967) showed that biceps acted for loads above 39 N.

Elbow flexion

The main elbow flexors are biceps, brachialis and brachioradialis (Basmajian and Latif, 1957), with less action in biceps if the limb is pronated and unloaded. Pauly, Rushing and Scheving (1967) reported similar findings, suggesting that brachioradialis acted mainly in fast movements. However, de Sousa, de Moraes and de Moraes Vieira (1961) found that brachioradialis was always active during flexion. Pronator teres was found to act as a flexor against resistance by Slaughter (1959), Basmajian and Travill (1961) and Pauly, Rushing and Scheving (1967). Slaughter noted that pronator teres continued to act as a flexor even when the forearm was simultaneously supinated, although to a lesser extent.

Elbow extension

The triceps is obviously the main elbow extensor, and has been studied electromyographically by Slaughter (1959), Travill (1962) and Pauly, Rushing and Scheving (1967). Travill noted that the medial head could act alone if there were no resistance to movement, that there was equal activity in both medial and lateral heads against moderate resistance, and that the long head was recruited last. Slaughter noted that the long head could remain quiescent if its action would oppose a simultaneous shoulder flexion movement. Pauly, Rushing and Scheving made no distinction between the three heads of triceps, noting that all three, plus anconeus, contracted simultaneously to extend the elbow against resistance. These authors, with Barnett and Harding (1955) and Basmajian (1967), noted that fast extension movements provoked a burst of protective reflex activity in the elbow flexors. This prevented hyperextension, with most activity in biceps.

The anconeus is generally agreed to be at least a minor elbow extensor, but various authors have also suggested that it aids forearm rotation. Basmajian and Griffin (1972) did not prove a definite function – it seems sensible to look on anconeus as an extension of the lateral head of triceps (Grant, 1947).

Forearm rotation

Both pronation and supination were examined by Travill and Basmajian (1961a, 1961b), who found that pronator quadratus and supinator acted alone when their respective rotations were not resisted. Pronator teres and biceps were recruited for rotations against resistance. Biceps action during supination was inhibited at full extension.

Other muscles have been suggested as accessory rotators, due to their slanting orientations in the forearm. The only conclusive finding has been that brachioradialis acted to produce rotations towards neutral from either extreme of rotation when such movements were resisted (Basmajian and Latif, 1957; Pauly, Rushing and Scheving, 1967).

Wrist and hand actions

It is important to note the actions of muscles which move and stabilize the wrist and hand because many of them originate from the humerus and therefore contribute to elbow joint forces. Backdahl and Carlsoo (1961) found that wrist movements were caused by exactly those muscles which one would predict: the flexors and extensors carpi radialis and ulnaris, with wrist flexion and extension assisted by flexor digitorum superficialis and extensor digitorum communis, respectively. These actions are in marked contrast to the activity seen when the hand is loaded. Long et al (1970) found graded increasing participation, in proportion to the loading, in all the extrinsic muscles except abductor pollicis longus, in all forms of power grip, presumably to stabilize the loaded hand on the forearm. Similarly, Dempster and Finerty (1947) found marked antagonistic actions to stabilize the wrist if the forearm was held horizontally in various rotations and the hand loaded vertically.

Elbow strength

Data presented in this section is of direct use for calculating the forces applied to the elbow joint.

Flexion

Many workers have published data on elbow flexion strength because it is a convenient site for investigation of muscle mechanics. The most comprehensive surveys of maximal elbow flexion strength, exerted isometrically, have been by Clarke et al (1950) and Hunsicker

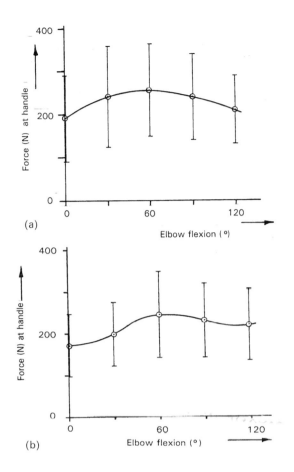

(a)

(b)

Figure 9.9 (a) Maximum elbow flexion strength at various elbow positions. (From Hunsicker, 1955.) (b) Maximum elbow extension strength at various elbow positions. (From Hunsicker, 1955.) Mean ± standard deviation.

(1955). Both studies used young male subjects and produced similar results, with a peak at 60° flexion (Figure 9.9a). The large standard deviations shown from Hunsicker's mean curve reveal the spread of strength in the population tested. Other studies have been less useful, either because the tests have been on small samples, or at a limited range of postures, or because of lack of subject restraint during the tests. If the subject is not adequately braced, then submaximal data will result – Hugh-Jones (1947) showed that strength when pulling on a lever was increased 70% by providing a foot rest. Arm strength is also influenced greatly by speed of movement: the tension–length curves of muscles being raised by a forced elongation against maximal contraction (eccentric loading condition) and reduced as the speed of con-

traction increases (Hill, 1951; Elftman, 1966). This was demonstrated at the elbow by Doss and Karpovich (1965), who produced elbow flexion strength curves with concentric force 23% smaller, and eccentric force 14% greater, than isometric strength. Hill (1951) found that the force generated to resist an applied stretch may be twice the isometric strength, an effect which explains triceps avulsion fractures of the olecranon during falls on to the outstretched hand.

Male and female flexion strengths were compared by Elkins, Ledan and Wakim (1951), who found the mean female strength to be 55% of that of the males. The effect of different forearm rotation positions on flexion and extension strength was investigated by Provins and Salter (1955), who found that neutral rotation gave greatest strength and pronation least. Flexion strength in pronation was reduced significantly when using a handle compared with use of a wrist cuff, suggesting that finger strength limited this action.

Extension

Isometric extension strength data has been published by Elkins, Ledan and Wakim (1951), Hunsicker (1955), Provins and Salter (1955) and Currier (1972). Maximum extension strength was found at 90° flexion by Elkins, Ledan and Wakim (1951) and Currier (1972), while a peak at 60° flexion was reported by Hunsicker (1955) and Provins and Salter (1955). The results of Hunsicker are presented for use (Figure 9.9b), partly because they were obtained from a large number of subjects, but primarily because they were significantly larger than those of other investigators, which suggests a lack of subject restraint in other investigations.

Forearm rotation

Forearm rotation strength was explored in detail by Darcus (1951) and Salter and Darcus (1952), using a handgrip dynamometer. The main finding, shown in Figure 9.10, was that a linear relationship existed between torque and position for both pronation and supination. The pronation torque increased as the forearm moved towards supination, i.e. as the pronation muscles were stretched, and a similar effect occurred with supination. The slope of the

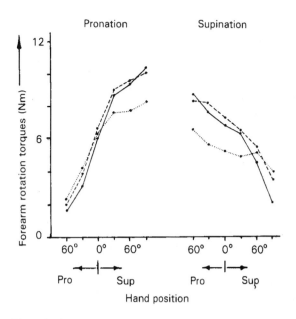

Figure 9.10 Forearm rotation strength at different elbow flexion angles: ———— 30°; – – – 90°; ...... 150° (From Darcus, 1951.)

pronation graph is steeper than for supination, reaching a higher peak value, and higher at the mid-position. It can be seen that elbow flexion had little effect on forearm rotation strength until 150° flexion. A similar procedure investigated the effect of shoulder position on rotation strength, which was tested with the shoulder adducted to the side of the body, flexed 90°, or abducted 90°. There was little effect when the elbow was maintained at 90° flexion.

Pulling

This strong action is limited by posture. Dempster (1958) showed that a load equal to the subject's body weight could be taken by each hand. Interestingly, when lifting, the force vector always passed posteriorly to the slightly flexed elbow, indicating a preponderance of triceps activity in such actions. A similar strength was reported by Hunsicker (1955): 530 ± 150 N standard deviation with the elbow extended and declining 25% with 90° flexion.

Pushing

Maximal loads can be applied along the forearm by pushing when braced against a back rest. Both Hugh-Jones (1947) and Hun-

sicker (1955) found that pushing strength increased towards full extension, peaking at 590 ± 150 N as the elbow 'toggled' into full extension.

Abduction and adduction

Hunsicker (1955) showed that these actions were relatively weak and remained approximately constant throughout the range of flexion. These actions cause torsion loads in the distal humerus, with associated collateral ligament tensions, when the elbow is flexed 90°. At 90° flexion, Hunsicker reported a mean abduction force of 156 ± 81 N and a mean adduction force of 218 ± 100 N when the hand was applied to a handle.

Strength of patients with rheumatoid arthritis

The great majority of elbow joint replacements will be for patients with rheumatoid arthritis, who are likely to place lesser demands than normal on their joints. Amis et al (1979a) studied isometric flexion strength, at 90° flexion, in 102 rheumatoid patients. Force was applied using a wide strap over the wrist, in 30° supination, a posture found to be comfortable by the rheumatoid patient. Male and female outpatients had mean strengths of 146 ± 76 and 57 ± 41 N, while values for male and female inpatients were 98 ± 46 and 57 ± 41 N, respectively. Since normal young adult strength is 228 N and 125 N for males and females, it is apparent that the average rheumatoid strength was 45% of normal. With a mean patient age of 55 years, some of this decrease was due to ageing, rather than the rheumatoid disease. It was felt that the findings for these rheumatoid patients would be representative for joint replacement candidates because the group measured included some whose elbows were nearly normal and others who had gross destruction.

Elbow joint forces

Since it was noted, in the introduction, that the muscles must work at a great mechanical disadvantage compared with the lever arms of external loads on the hand, it follows that the muscle actions will dominate the joint forces.

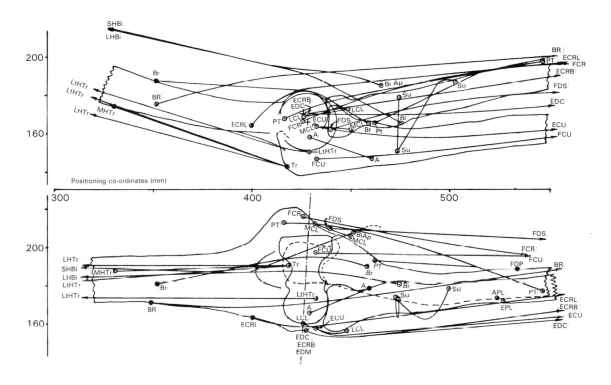

Figure 9.11 The paths of the centroids of the muscle cross-sections in the region of the elbow. (From Amis, Dowson and Wright, 1979.)

Because of this, it is essential that any estimation of joint forces is based on an accurate assessment of which muscles contribute to the action being analysed, and also on an accurate knowledge of the musculoskeletal geometry, so that the lines of action of the muscles passing across the joint are known. The 'which muscles?' question can be answered by reference to the electromyographic data reviewed above, but further knowledge is required both to decide where the muscles act, in relation to the elbow axis in flexion and extension, and to decide how to apportion the co-operating actions of individual muscles contracting in groups. Early analyses simplified the muscle structures down to just two or three elbow flexors and one extensor, and apportioned their loads on the basis of their sizes (Groh, 1973; Walker, 1977). Since most elbow actions also involve grasping actions of the hand, and wrist stabilizing actions, it is apparent that allowance for the forearm muscle actions would both increase the elbow joint forces from those derived by simplified analyses and also predict that they acted in different directions.

Musculoskeletal data

Several approaches have been proposed to allow muscle actions to be estimated. Electromyographic outputs from muscles can be related to their tensions (Hof and van den Berg, 1977), but not easily in sufficient detail for this purpose. Also, mathematical optimization criteria have been tried (Seireg and Arvikar, 1973; Penrod, Davy and Singh, 1974), but these have little practical confirmation beyond their ability to conform to electromyographic findings. Other workers have sought to relate the strengths of individual muscles to their physical dimensions, such as cross-sectional area (Ikai and Fukunaga, 1968). This was developed further by Alexander and Vernon (1975), who derived formulae for the 'physiological cross-section' (PCS) that allowed for the pennated fibre orientation in some muscles. Pennation allows many fibres, in what may appear to be a long slim muscle, to slant across it from a tendon of origin to one of insertion, increasing the strength greatly but decreasing the contraction distance. This arrangement is seen in most

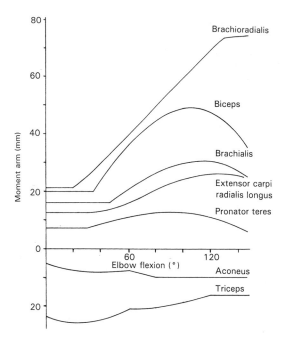

Figure 9.12 Moment arms for different elbow muscles during elbow movement.

of the forearm muscles. Knowledge of the PCS of each of a group of maximally contracting muscles allows forces to be shared between them, as they are all likely to be similarly stressed, and force equals stress × area. Alexander and Vernon obtained data to support this method from various species, including humans. Data for the PCSs of the upper limb muscles were published by Amis, Dowson and Wright (1979) and An et al (1981).

The three-dimensional geometry of the upper limb musculoskeletal system was obtained by measurement of the coordinates around muscle attachments and around individual muscles at the elbow and wrist of cadaveric preparations, leading to diagrams showing the paths of the centroids of the muscle cross-sections, as described by Jensen and Metcalf (1975) (Figure 9.11; Amis, Dowson and Wright, 1979). This information was manipulated to derive graphs of muscle moment arm variations with elbow flexion (Figure 9.12). The flexor muscles were found to have constant moment arms towards full extension as they rested on the anterior joint capsule. Comparison with the scant data previously available showed good agreement (Braune and Fischer, 1890; Haxton, 1945; Wilkie, 1949).

Joint forces in elbow flexion

This action, and subsequent actions, will be analysed with the forearm in neutral rotation to avoid extremes of muscle path or carrying angle. The electromyographic literature (above) has shown that all the elbow flexors are active, and the strength reports have also shown a maximum in this position.

Since flexion activities normally involve the hand in grasping and lifting an object, such as a handle, it is apparent that the forearm flexor muscles will contract (Long et al, 1970). Since this gripping action tends to flex the wrist, antagonistic extensor carpi muscle actions must stabilize the wrist. With the forearm flexing in neutral rotation, the external load pulls towards ulnar deviation of the wrist, and this must be resisted by biasing the wrist stabilizers towards a radial deviation action. This is a complex indeterminate situation, but fortunately Dempster and Finerty (1947) produced comprehensive data on stabilization of the wrist against transverse forces by using electromyographic studies. The forces assigned to the forearm muscles were primarily in proportion to their PCSs, but were scaled down in accordance with Dempster and Finerty, providing the correct actions to resist the external load. The main action was found to be in the extensor carpi radialis muscles, which stabilize the wrist against both flexion and ulnar deviation actions. Since these muscles cross the elbow at the lateral side, it is not surprising that wrist stabilization alone was predicted to cause humero-radial joint forces in excess of four times the external load applied to the hand. Since only part of the finger flexor action crosses the humero-ulnar joint, via flexor digitorum superficialis, the humero-ulnar joint force due to gripping was predicted to be only 0.4 of the external force. Because the majority of the wrists flexors and extensors originate close to the flexion axis of the elbow (extensor carpi radialis longus passes anterior to the axis, causing flexion), hand gripping and wrist stabilizing efforts have a very small effect on elbow flexion–extension equilibrium.

The flexor muscle forces necessary to resist the external moment were found by scaling them up until equilibrium was obtained, with their relative contributions according to their sizes (PCSs). This meant that they were all assumed to have an equal stress acting on their

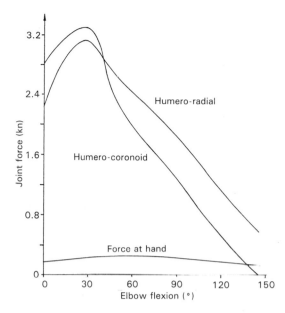

Figure 9.13 The joint forces calculated to act at the elbow joint during flexion.

fibres in this maximal isometric loading. After doing this, forearm rotation equilibrium was examined, and it was found that pronator teres imposed a larger rotation moment than the opposing biceps tension when their tensions had been assigned according to their PCSs. Pronator teres was therefore relaxed to obtain rotation equilibrium. A final touch was to apply a stabilizing action to the joint, and a triceps tension was imposed, equal to 18% of biceps tension, as suggested by Messier et al (1971).

The muscle forces became: biceps 6.4, brachialis 6.2, pronator teres 3.2 and brachioradialis 1.9 times the external force at the fully extended position.

Since three of the flexors insert into the radius, it is not surprising that flexion causes large humero-radial joint forces. An anterior view of the forearm shows that biceps and pronator teres tend to pull the radius into varus. This is resisted, via the distal radioulnar joint, by compressive force on the large medial lip of the trochlea. Calculations following the above scheme were performed using muscle path geometry data corresponding to a range of elbow flexion angles, with the external force acting on the hand in accordance with the data for maximum isometric strength detailed above. Figures 9.13 and 9.14 show that large forces were predicted to act on both humero-radial and humero-ulnar joints during flexion. The joint forces are a much greater multiple of the external load on the hand near full extension because the flexor muscles then lie close to the elbow flexion axis and so have a large 'mechanical disadvantage' to overcome. It is seen that the forces are effectively on to the end of the humerus when the elbow is extended, and swing round to act on the anterior aspect as the elbow flexes. The antero-posterior force component is demonstrated graphically in the clinic because loosened humeral prosthesis components tend to migrate posteriorly (Souter, 1977). The joint forces during flexion are always predicted to act within the bounds of the

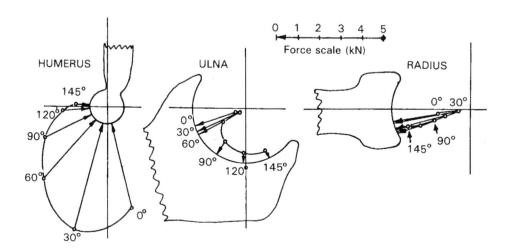

Figure 9.14 The sagittal plane forces acting on the different parts of the elbow joint. Note the radius and ulna transmit similar forces.

articular surfaces of both radius and ulna, normally in a distal and slightly posterior direction which is towards the base of the coronoid process and towards the posterior rim of the radial head. Thus subluxation will not normally occur and onlay type prosthetic components should function satisfactorily. Although Figure 9.14 presents only the forces acting in the sagittal plane, the force analysis from which these results were derived was fully three-dimensional. This was particularly necessary for understanding the equilibrium of the radius, which is effectively like a tent pole on top of a ball, maintained by the muscle tensions acting like guy ropes. The muscles act predominantly in the sagittal plane, so it is not surprising that radioulnar joint forces are trivially small at approximately 10% of the humero-ulnar force. This action arises largely from the slanting orientation of pronator teres. The dominant finding was that the radius and ulna were predicted to transmit similar loads to the humerus – the elbow acts as a bicondylar joint.

Forces in extension

With the neutral forearm rotation posture used, this action required an ulnar abduction effort at the wrist. Since wrist extensor action was required to maintain the equilibrium of the hand against the flexion moment caused by gripping, the predominant effect was to load extensor carpi ulnaris. This helped to transfer forces from the ulna to the radius at the elbow, which is beneficial because of the very large triceps force acting on the ulna in extension. A further factor that transfers force from ulna to radius in this situation is that the powerful lateral head of triceps dissipates partly into fascia overlying the supinator muscle. Use of the data on muscle strength and moment arms, and the equal-stress criterion, gave the following forces: triceps main tendon 11.5 N, lateral head force passing to radius 2 N, anconeus force 0.6 N, per unit of force at the hand, at 0° flexion. This procedure was repeated at points throughout the range of flexion, with a stabilizing biceps tension of 7% of triceps tension, as suggested by Messier et al (1971). The biceps rotation effect was assumed to be balanced by pronator quadratus, which would also act to maintain compression of the distal radioulnar joint against the triceps action.

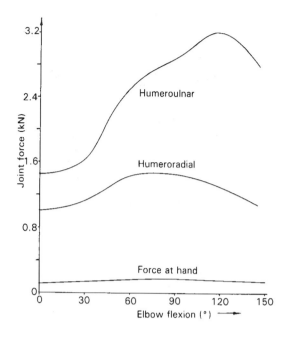

Figure 9.15 The joint forces calculated to act at the elbow joint during extension.

The results of the equilibrium calculations were then multiplied up in line with the published extension strength data to give the joint forces shown in Figure 9.15. The most important finding, as expected, was the size of the humero-ulnar force, 3.2 kN, arising from the triceps tendon tension reaching almost 3 kN. Although this is a stable situation with the joint force acting into the floor of the trochlear notch of the ulna, a large tensile stress is caused in the bone of the olecranon. It is not surprising that the olecranon is fractured during falls, as a forced stretch of the triceps will raise its tension above the isometric value noted above, leading to avulsion failure. If the bone survives this effect during a fall, the impact of the posterior aspect of the elbow on to the ground may then cause fracture with little further trauma. It follows that the designer of an elbow prosthesis should ensure that the prosthetic component and its implantation procedure will not require unnecessary excavation of the olecranon, particularly since it is usually eroded from both sides by the rheumatoid disease.

Forces when pulling

At first sight a large tension load on the upper

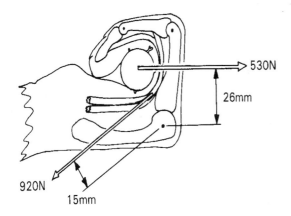

Figure 9.16 The forces generated at the hand during pulling or lifting.

limb, such as occurs when lifting a heavy suitcase, seems a likely mechanism for loosening a joint replacement (Lee and Ling, 1977). However, analysis of the mechanics of pulling actions shows that the joints of the upper limb are actually *compressed* by muscle actions which overcome the external load. This arises primarily because of the geometry of the fingers during gripping actions such as the 'suitcase pull' (Napier, 1956), when the flexor tendon tensions are approximately twice the external load.

The geometry of the situation is shown in Figure 9.16, a sagittal section through a ring finger flexed into a hook grip. Consideration of the flexion–extension equilibrium of the metacarpophalangeal joint shows that the external load has a moment arm of 26 mm, while the tendons of flexors digitorum profundus and superficialis pass approximately 15 mm from the joint axis, Thus, for a pulling force of 530 N, the tendons will have a combined tension of 920 N, leaving 390 N to compress the wrist. This is not all, however, because the wrist is stabilized by simultaneous actions of many of the forearm muscles (Long et al, 1970), which will add to the compressive force. Analysis of wrist stability allows these muscle forces to be predicted, leading to a wrist compressive force of 1180 N. Since much of the finger flexor tendon tension is transmitted to the radius, ulna and interosseous membrane, only a part of the wrist compressive force acts across the elbow joint line. The resultant has been calculated to be a force of 210 N compressing each of the radial head and coronoid process.

In view of the above prediction, it seems likely that elbow prostheses will not be subjected to tensile forces acting on their fixations.

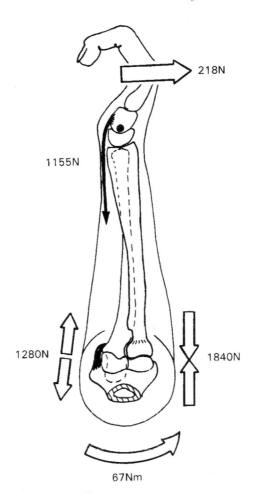

Figure 9.17 Active forearm adduction with the elbow flexed to 90°; large rotational forces occur, which will tend to cause prosthesis loosening.

It is possible that tensile forces could arise if a load is suspended from a wrist strap, thus avoiding the need for forearm muscle actions. This situation is analogous to the circumstance in which small children suffer from a 'pulled elbow', where the radial head is distracted from the annular ligament after the arm is pulled suddenly when the forearm muscles are relaxed.

Forearm adduction with the elbow flexed to 90°

This movement might place considerable strain on the elbow. It would occur when the palms of the hands are pressed inwards on the sides of a box held in front of the body. The force at the hands arises from a large inward rotation torque applied to the humerus by the pectoral muscles. With the force acting on to the palm of the hand, the finger muscles need only contribute to wrist stabilization. Comparison of the moment arms of the external force and wrist flexor tendons about the centre of the wrist (Figure 9.17) shows that a trans-wrist tendon force of four times the external load is needed for equilibrium. Allowance for the antagonistic stabilizing actions described by Dempster and Finerty (1947) raises this to 5.3 times the external load, of which 2.6 N per 1 N of external force passes across the elbow.

The equilibrium of the elbow is examined by taking moments about the centre of the capitellum. The external force has a large moment arm so, despite the muscle tension crossing the joint, the coronoid tends to lift off the trochlea and valgus opening is resisted by the medial collateral ligament tension of 5.9 N per unit force at the hand. Thus the humero-radial joint force is 5.9 N ligament tension plus 2.6 N muscle tension, or 8.5 times the external load. Hunsicker (1955) reported an average male strength of 218 N (a humeral torque of 67 Nm), giving a humeroradial force of 1.84 kN and a medial collateral ligament tension of 1.28 kN, with no humeroulnar loading.

The above results show the advantage of the width of the distal humerus, the distance from the capitellum to the medial epicondyle increasing the lever or moment arm of the ligament and hence decreasing its tension. Elbow prostheses which do not utilize this tissue structure inevitably magnify the forces on their fixations as these concentrate close to the axis of the humerus. This applied particularly to the early designs of 'hinge arthroplasty' (Souter, 1973).

Forearm abduction, with the elbow flexed to 90°

In this situation the fingers take up a hook grip, as though tearing an object apart. This means that there are finger flexor tendon tensions acting to flex the wrist, as well as the action of the external load. A large extensor carpi action was therefore needed, in order to stabilize the wrist, which was predicted to be large enough to compress the humero-radial joint despite the action of the external load. This, of course, meant that the forearm was stable against the varus action of the load without a lateral collateral ligament tension. Hunsicker (1955) reported a mean strength of 156 N (a humeral external rotation torque of 48 Nm), leading to a humero-radial force of 0.7 kN, a humero-

ulnar force of 1.65 kN and a wrist force of 2.76 kN.

These results are an interesting contrast to those seen during adduction, when the medial collateral ligament was tensed. This difference in behaviour arises primarily because all the major wrist extensors cross the elbow, compressing the radial head, whereas flexor digitorum profundus and the majority of flexor carpi ulnaris do not. These predictions appear to be reasonable when the collateral ligament structures are compared. The medial ligament has a substantial anterior band, the primary stabilizer of the elbow (Schwab et al, 1980; Miller, 1981), whereas the lateral collateral structure dissipates into the annular ligament and tendinous edge of the anconeus and does not locate the radius in as stable a position as does the medial ligament.

Axial loads on the forearm and radial head excision

There are two main sources of axial loading on the bones of the forearm: external forces acting on the hand, and internal muscle actions, which have been analysed above. The external forces may arise during voluntary pushing actions, or from impacts caused by falling on to the outstretched hand. A matter of particular concern is the role of the head of radius, which

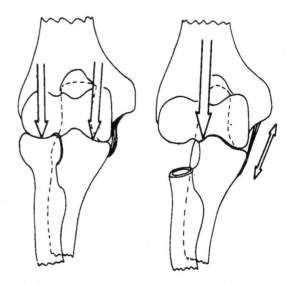

Figure 9.18 After radial head excision large medial collateral ligament forces are predicted, causing the elbow to drift into valgus.

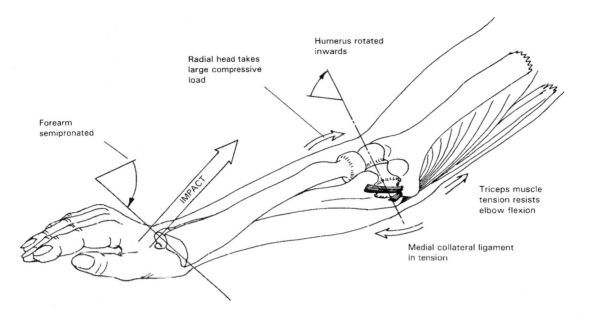

Forearm
semipronated

Radial head takes
large compressive
load

Humerus rotated
inwards

IMPACT

Triceps muscle
tension resists
elbow flexion

Medial collateral ligament
in tension

Figure 9.19 The usual situation with a fall on to the outstretched hand.

has been shown previously to sustain large forces in many activities, causing the elbow to function as a balanced bicondylar articulation. Excision of the head of the radius is controversial, but is widely accepted as part of the surgical treatment of rheumatoid arthritis in conjunction with synovectomy (Laine and Vainio, 1969; Taylor, Mukerjea and Rana, 1976). This procedure is also accepted practice after comminuted fractures of the radial head, but some authors have reported a significant rate of disabling wrist symptoms in such cases (Lewis and Thibodeau, 1937; McDougall and White, 1957; Taylor and O'Connor, 1964). Wrist symptoms have been linked to the degree of use of the limb, and it has been suggested that disruption of the distal radioulnar joint results from stretching of the interosseous membrane. The fibres of the membrane are largely arranged so that forces acting to push the radius proximally can be resisted by their tension acting distally towards their origins on the ulna. It was suggested by Amis et al (1979b) that radial head excision would cause the humero-radial joint forces to be transferred to the humero-ulnar joint, and that a large medial collateral ligament tension would be needed to prevent valgus angulation (Figure 9.18). This increase in the carrying angle has been reported after radial head excision in trauma (Taylor and O'Connor, 1964) and in rheumatoid disease

(Rymaszewski et al, 1984).

The transmission of external force from the hand to the elbow was studied by Halls and Travill (1964), who suggested that the radius transmitted 50–70% of the load directly from the hand to the humerus. This certainly ties in with the observation that the hand is supported mainly by the radius, and that the radius develops as a compression strut. A similar result was described by Walker (1977), although he felt that little force reached the capitellum below 100 N (but this finding was probably due to artefact). One drawback of the reports of these researchers was that they used a fixed alignment of their specimens, with an axial force. An analysis of the realistic situation shows that impact forces during falls do not pass neatly along the forearm, but that the forearm is always rotated to load the humero-radial joint in compression, and tense the medial collateral ligament (Figure 9.19). Carlsoo and Johansson (1962) studied voluntary falls on to the outstretched hand and noted simultaneous contraction of both biceps and triceps bracing the elbow with at least 15° flexion before impact. The force was diminished by a controlled collapse of the elbow, dissipating the energy by stretching the triceps.

The experiments of Amis et al (1981) applied loads to the hand or distal radius in different directions, axially and then with valgus and

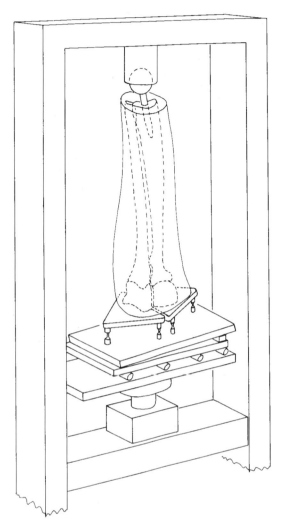

Figure 9.20 Loading the elbow in an experiment in the laboratory.

The role of the interosseous membrane was examined after radial head excision. Axial forces caused the forearm to move into valgus above 100 N. The membrane was found to have a stiffness of approximately 200 N/mm, which was much lower than the 1400 N/mm of the humero-radial joint. This means that the radius may well be displaced proximally by muscle actions in the strenuous activities analysed above, disrupting the distal radio-ulnar joint. Furthermore, the stiffnesses of the structures mean that only one-eighth of any axial load is transmitted by the membrane when the head of radius is present. It seems that the primary purpose of the slanting fibres in the membrane is to act as an origin for the deep flexor muscles of the forearm, channelling their forces to the radiocarpal joint rather than the head of ulna and overlying triangular fibrocartilage. The biomechanical analysis suggests that radial head excision should not be undertaken lightly and that prosthetic replacement of the radial head should be considered for active patients.

Conclusion

The biomechanics of the elbow are complex, but this review highlights the large forces which occur in the region of the elbow. These forces will tend to cause loosening and failure of elbow prostheses. Modern prosthesis design must be tailored to reducing this risk of loosening and failure by providing the best mechanical advantage for the bone–prosthesis interface.

References

Alexander RMcN and Vernon A (1975) The dimensions of knee and ankle muscles and the forces they exert. *Journal of Human Movement Studies* **1** 115–123.

American Academy of Orthopedic Surgeons (1966) *Joint Motion: Method of Measuring and Recording*, 97 pp. Edinburgh: Churchill Livingstone.

Amis AA (1978) Biomechanics of the upper limb, and design of an elbow prosthesis. PhD Thesis, Leeds University.

Amis AA & Miller JH (1982) The elbow. *Clinics in Rheumatic Diseases* **8** 571–593.

Amis AA, Dowson D and Wright V (1979) Elbow joint force predictions for some strenuous isometric actions. *Journal of Biomechanics* **13** 765–775.

Amis AA, Dowson D, Unsworth A, Miller JH and Wright

varus angulations. The forces transmitted to the capitellum and trochlea were measured directly by mounting the separated humeral condyles on to adjacent force plates and then loading the entire assembly in a compression test machine (Figure 9.20). It was found that the forearm remained stable on the humerus when the force path passed through the humeroradial joint, with 73% of the load passing to the capitellum at all loads up to 1.2 kN. Varus or valgus angulation caused the specimen to collapse if the force path was outside the width of the joint, indicating collateral ligament tension in vivo, with 100% of the axial load acting on to the coronoid in varus and on to the radial head in valgus.

V (1977) An examination of the elbow articulation with particular reference to variation of the carrying angle. *Engineering in Medicine* **6** 76–80.

Amis AA, Hughes S, Miller JH, Wright V and Dowson D (1979a) Elbow joint forces in patients with rheumatoid arthritis. *Rheumatology and Rehabilitation* **18** 230–234.

Amis AA, Miller JH, Dowson D and Wright V (1979b) Biomechanical aspects of the elbow: joint forces related to prosthesis design. *Journal of Medical Engineering and Technology* **3** 229–234.

Amis AA, Miller JH, Dowson D and Wright V (1981) Axial forces in the forearm: their relationship to excision of the head of radius. In *Mechanical Factors and the Skeleton* (IAF Stokes, ed.), pp. 29–37. London: Libbey.

Amis AA, Hughes S, Miller, JH, Wright V and Dowson D (1982) A functional study of the rheumatoid elbow. *Rheumatology and Rehabilitation* **21** 151–157.

An KN, Hui FC, Morrey BF, Linscheid RL and Chao EY (1981) Muscles across the elbow joint: a biomechanical analysis. *Journal of Biomechanics* **14** 659–669.

Backdahl M and Carlsoo S (1961) Distribution of activity in muscles acting on the wrist (an electromyographic study). *Acta Morphologica Neerlando-Scandinavica* **4** 136–144.

Barnett CH and Harding D (1955) The activity of antagonist muscles during voluntary movements. *Annals of Physical Medicine* **2** 290–293.

Barter JT, Emanuel I and Truett B. (1957) *A statistical evaluation of joint range data.* Report No. WADC-TN-57-311. Ohio: Wright Air Development Center, Wright–Patterson Air Force Base.

Basmajian JV (1967) *Muscles Alive*, 2nd edn. Baltimore: Williams and Wilkins

Basmajian JV and Griffin WR (1972) Function of anconeus muscle – an electromyographic study. *Journal of Bone and Joint Surgery* **54A** 1712–1714.

Basmajian JV and Latif A (1957) Integrated actions and functions of the chief flexors of the elbow. *Journal of Bone and Joint Surgery* **39A** 1106–1118.

Basmajian JV and Travill AA (1961) Electromyography of the pronator muscles in the forearm. *Anatomical Record* **139** 45–49.

Boone DC and Azen SP (1979) Normal range of motion of joints in male subjects. *Journal of Bone and Joint Surgery* **61A** 756–759.

Braune W and Fischer O (1890) Die Rotationsmomente der Beugemuskeln am Ellenbogengelenk des Menschen, *Abh. d. konigl.-sachs. Ges. Wiss. Mathem-Phys.* K1.15., cited by Groh (1973).

Burrough SJ (1973) The design of an elbow prosthesis, *Engineering in Medicine* **2** 64–67.

Capener N (1956) The hand in surgery. *Journal of Bone and Joint Surgery* **38B** 128–151.

Carlsoo S and Johansson O (1962) Stabilisation of, and load on, the elbow joint in some protective movements. *Acta Anatomica Scandinavica* **48** 224–231.

Cave EF and Roberts SM (1936) A method for ensuring and recording joint function. *Journal of Bone and Joint Surgery* **18** 455–465.

Chao EY, An KN, Askew LJ and Morrey BF (1980) Electrogoniometer for the measurement of human elbow joint rotation. *Journal of Biomechanical Engineering* **102** 301.

Clark WA (1920) A system of joint measurements. *Journal of Orthopaedic Surgery* **2** 687–700.

Clarke HH, Elkins EC, Wakim KG and Martin GM (1950) Relationship between body position and the application of muscle power to movements of the joints. *Archives of Physical Medicine and Rehabilitation* **31** 81–89.

Currier DP (1972) Maximal isometric tension of the elbow extensors at varied positions. *Physical Therapy* **52** 1043–1049.

Darcus HD (1951) The maximum torques developed in pronation and supination of the right hand. *Journal of Anatomy* **85** 55–67.

Darcus HD and Salter N (1953) The amplitude of pronation and supination with the elbow flexed to a right angle. *Journal of Anatomy* **87** 169–184.

Dempster WT (1955) *Space requirements of the seated operator. Geometrical, kinematic, and mechanical aspects of the body with special reference to the limbs.* Project No. 7214. Ohio: Wright Air Development Center, Wright–Patterson Air Force Base.

Dempster WT (1958) Analysis of two-handed pulls using free-body diagrams. *Journal of Applied Physiology* **13** 469–480.

Dempster WT and Finerty JC (1947) Relative activity of wrist moving muscles in static support of the wrist joint: an electromyographic study. *American Journal of Physiology* **150** 596–606.

de Sousa OM, de Moraes JL and de Moraes Vieira FL (1961) Electromyographic study of the brachioradialis muscle. *Anatomical Record* **139** 125–131.

Doss WS and Karpovich PV (1965) A comparison of concentric, eccentric, and isometric strength of elbow flexors. *Journal of Applied Physiology* **20** 351–353.

Dwight T (1884) The movements of the ulna in rotation of the forearm. *Journal of Anatomy and Physiology* **19** 186–189.

Elftman H (1966) Biomechanics of muscle. *Journal of Bone and Joint Surgery* **48A** 363–377.

Elkins EC, Ledan UM and Wakim KG (1951) Objective recording of the strength of normal muscles. *Archives of Physical Medicine* **32** 639–647.

Ewald FC (1975) Total elbow replacement. *Orthopedic Clinics of North America* **6** 685–696.

Fick R (1911) *Spezielle Gelenk- und Muskelmechanik*, pp. 284–399. Jena: G Fisher.

Fischer O (1907) *Kinematik Organischer Gelenke*. Braunschweig: F Vierweg.

Glanville AD and Kreezer G (1937) The maximum amplitude and velocity of joint movements in normal male human adults. *Human Biology* **9** 197–211.

Goodfellow JW and Bullough PG (1967) The pattern of ageing of the articular cartilage of the elbow joint. *Journal of Bone and Joint Surgery* **49B** 175–181.

Grant JCB (1947) *An Atlas of Anatomy*, 2nd edn. Baltimore: Williams and Wilkins.

Groh H (1973) Proceedings I Elbow Fractures in the adult I. General (a) Anatomy biomechanics of the elbow joint. *Hefte zu Unfallheilkund* **114** 13–20.

Halls AA and Travill A (1964) Transmission of pressures across the elbow joint. *Anatomical Record* **150** 243–247.

Haxton H (1945) A comparison of the action of extension of the knee and elbow joints in man. *Anatomical Record* **93** 279–286.

Heiberg J (1884) The movements of the ulna in rotation of the forearm. *Journal of Anatomy and Physiology* **19** 237–240.

Hertzberg HTE (1972) Engineering anthropology. In *Human Engineering Guide to Equipment Design* (HP Cott and RG Kinkade, eds), Washington: US Government Printing Office.

Hill AV (1951) The mechanics of voluntary muscle. *Lancet* **261** 947–951.

Hof AL and van den Berg JW (1977) Linearity between the weighted sums of the emg's of the human triceps surae and the total torque. *Journal of Biomechanics* **10** 529–539.

Hugh-Jones P (1947) The effect of limb position in seated subjects on their ability to utilise the maximum contractile force of the limb muscles. *Journal of Physiology* **104** 332–344.

Hultkrantz JW (1897) *Das Ellbogengelenk und seine Mechanik.* Munich: Jena.

Hunsicker P (1955) *Arm strength at selected degrees of elbow flexion.* Technical Report 54-548. Ohio: Wright Air Development Centre, Wright–Patterson Air Force Base.

Ikai M and Fukunaga T (1986) Calculations of muscle strength per unit of cross-sectional area of human muscle by means of ultrasonic measurement. *Int. Z. angew. Physiol. einschi. Arbeitsphysiol* **26** 26–32.

Jensen RH and Metcalf WK (1975) A systematic approach to the quantitative description of musculo-skeletal geometry. *Journal of Anatomy* **119** 209–221.

Kapandji IA (1970) *The Physiology of the Joints*, 2nd edn, vol. 1: Upper Limb. Edinburgh: Livingstone.

Laine V and Vainio K (1969) Synovectomy of the elbow. In *Early Synovectomy in RA* (W Hijmans, WD Paul and H Herschel, eds), pp. 117–118 Amsterdam: Exerpta Medica.

Lee AJC and Ling RSM (1977) The optimised use of pmma bone cement and some limitations of its use in the fixation of upper limb prostheses. In *Joint Replacement in the Upper Limb*, pp. 41–44 London: Institution of Mechanical Engineers.

Lewis RW and Thibodeau AA (1937) Deformity of the wrist following resection of the radial head. *Surgery, Gynecology and Obstetrics* **64** 1079–1085.

London JT (1981) Kinematics of the elbow. *Journal of Bone and Joint Surgery* **63A** 529–535.

Long C, Conrad PW, Hall EA and Furler SL (1970) Intrinsic–extrinsic muscle control of the hand in power grip and precision handling. An electromyographic study. *Journal of Bone and Joint Surgery* **53A** 853–867.

McDougall A and White J (1957) Subluxation of inferior radio-ulnar joint complicating fracture of radial head. *Journal of Bone and Joint Surgery* **39B** 278–287.

Messier RH, Duffey J, Litchman HM, Pasley PR, Soechting JF and Stewart PA (1971) The electromyogram as a measure of tension in the human biceps and triceps muscles. *International Journal of Mechanical Science* **13** 585–598.

Miller JH (1981) Mechanism of elbow injuries. In *An Introduction to the Biomechanics of Joints and Joint Replacement* (D Dowson and V Wright eds), pp. 222–234. London: Mechanical Engineering Publications.

Morrey BF and Chao EYS (1976) Passive motion of the elbow joint: a biomechanical analysis. *Journal of Bone and Joint Surgery* **58A** 501–508.

Napier JR (1956) The prehensile movements of the human hand. *Journal of Bone and Joint Surgery* **38B** 902–913.

Nicol AC (1977) Elbow joint prosthesis design: biomechanical aspects. PhD Thesis, University of Strathclyde, Glasgow.

Patrick J (1946) A study of supination and pronation with special reference to the treatment of forearm fractures. *Journal of Bone and Joint Surgery* **28B** 737–748.

Pauly JE, Rushing JL and Scheving LE (1967) An electromyographic study of some muscles crossing the elbow joint. *Anatomical Record* **159** 47–54.

Penrod DD, Davy DT and Singh DP (1974) An optimisation approach to tendon force analysis. *Journal of Biomechanics* **7** 123–129.

Potter HP (1895) The obliquity of the arm of the female in extension. The relation of the forearm with the upper arm in flexion. *Journal of Anatomy and Physiology* **29** 488–491.

Provins KA and Salter N (1955) Maximum torque exerted about the elbow joint *Journal of Applied Physiology* **7** 393–398.

Ray RD, Johnson RJ and Jameson RM (1951) Rotation of the forearm: an experimental study of pronation and supination. *Journal of Bone and Joint Surgery* **33A** 993–996.

Rymaszewski LA, Mackay I, Amis AA and Miller JH (1984) Long term effects of radial head excision in rheumatoid arthritis. *Journal of Bone and Joint Surgery* **66B** 109–113.

Salter N and Darcus HD (1952) The effect of the degree of elbow flexion on the maximum torques developed in pronation and supination of the right hand. *Journal of Anatomy* **86** 197–202.

Salter N and Darcus HD (1953) The amplitude of forearm and of humeral rotation. *Journal of Anatomy* **87** 407–418.

Schwab GH, Bennet JB, Woods GW and Tullos HS (1980) Biomechanics of elbow instability: the role of the medial collateral ligament. *Clinical Orthopaedics* **146** 42–52.

Seedhom BB and Tsubuku M (1977) A technique for the study of contact between visco-elastic bodies with special reference to the patello-femoral joint *Journal of Biomechanics* **10** 253–260.

Seedhom BB, Dowson D, Wright V and Longton EB (1973) A technique for the study of geometry and contact of natural and artificial knee joints. *Wear* **6** 189–199.

Seireg A and Arvikar RJ (1973) Mathematical model for evaluation of the forces in the lower extremities of the musculo-skeletal system. *Journal of Biomechanics* **6** 313–326.

Silverman S, Constine L, Harvey W and Grahame R (1975) Survey of joint mobility and in-vivo skin elasticity in London schoolchildren. *Annals of the Rheumatic Diseases* **34** 177–180.

Sinelnikoff E and Grigorowitsch M (1931) Die Bewegligkeit der Gelenke als sckundares geschlechtliches und konstitutionelles Merkmal. *Abteilung 2. Zeitschrift für Konstitutionslehre* **15** 679 cited by Hertzberg (1972).

Slaughter DR (1959) Electromyographic studies of arm movements. *Research Quarterly* **30** 326–337.

Smith L (1960) Deformity following supracondylar fractures of the humerus. *Journal of Bone and Joint Surgery* **42A** 235–252.

Sorbie C, Shiba R, Siu D, Saunders G and Wevers H (1986) The development of a surface arthroplasty for the elbow. *Clinical Orthopaedics* **208** 100–103.

Souter WA (1973) Arthroplasty of the elbow with particular reference to metallic hinge arthroplasty in rheumatoid patients. *Orthopedic Clinics of North America* **4** 395–413.

Souter WA (1977) Total replacement arthroplasty of the elbow. In *Joint Replacement in the Upper Limb*, pp. 99–106. London: Institution of Mechanical Engineers.

Steindler A (1964) *Kinesiology of the Human Body under Normal and Pathological Conditions*, 2nd edn. Springfield, IL: Thomas.

Street DM and Stevens PS (1974) A humeral replacement prosthesis for the elbow. *Journal of Bone and Joint Surgery* **56A** 1147–1158.

Taylor AR, Mukerjea SK and Rana NA (1976) Excision of the head of the radius in rheumatoid arthritis. *Journal of Bone and Joint Surgery* **58B** 485–487.

Taylor CL and Blaschke AC (1948) A method for kinematic analysis of motions of the shoulder, arm, and hand complex. *Annals of the New York Academy of Sciences* **51** 1251–1265.

Taylor TKF and O'Connor BT (1964) The effect on inferior radio-ulnar joint of excision of head of radius in adults. *Journal of Bone and Joint Surgery* **46B** 83–88.

Travill AA (1962) Electromyographic study of the extensor apparatus of the forearm. *Anatomical Record* **144** 373–376.

Travill AA and Basmajian JV (1961a) Electromyography of the pronators of the forearm. *Anatomical Record* **139** 45–49.

Travill AA and Basmajian JV (1961b) Electromyography of the supinators of the forearm. *Anatomical Record* **139** 557–560.

Walker PS (1977) *Human Joints and their Artificial Replacements*. Springfield, IL: Thomas.

West CC (1945) Measurement of joint motion. *Archives of Physical Medicine* **26** 414 425.

Wilkie DR (1949) The relation between force and velocity in human muscle. *Journal of Physiology* **110** 249–280.

Yamaguchi B (1972) The bipartient tendency of the articular surface of the trochlear notch in the human ulna. *Okajimas Folia Anatomica Japonica* **49** 23–35.

Youm Y, Dryer RF, Thambyrajah K et al (1979) Biomechanical analyses of forearm pronation–supination and elbow flexion–extension. *Journal of Biomechanics* **12** 245–255.

Zimmer EA (1968) *Borderlands of the Normal and Early Pathologic in Skeletal Roentgenology*. New York: Grune and Stratton.

10

Total elbow replacement

W. Angus Wallace

Elbow replacement is one of the newer joint replacement procedures and only a limited number of orthopaedic surgeons have had the opportunity to gain experience in this field. Those who have developed expertise have been able to observe the many problems associated with this particular joint, and the more arthroplasties they carry out the more cautious they become. It is now becoming clearer to surgeons that elbow replacement should still be reserved for certain categories of patient and that the results from elbow replacement cannot currently emulate those of hip or knee replacement in the 1990s. It is also important that patients are educated in what is possible and what is not, because many have an unrealistic expectation, particularly knowing how successful hip and knee replacements have been in friends and relatives. The decision-making process must be carried out with caution and the surgeon must develop a good patient–doctor relationship before embarking on this form of surgery. This chapter will explore the pathological causes of a stiff painful elbow, the surgical options for treatment and the types of joint replacement implants that are available and which should be considered. Finally, the surgical techniques will be described, before discussion of the complications and their management.

Surgical options for the stiff painful elbow

Rheumatoid arthritis with joint stiffness with or without articular surface damage

Many patients with rheumatoid arthritis have elbow involvement and the majority can be managed with conservative measures: analgesics, non-steroidal anti-inflammatory drugs and occasionally physiotherapy. During acute episodes of inflammation night splintage will prevent progressive flexion deformities from developing. However, once a flexion deformity is present it can be difficult to manage conservatively. Experienced physiotherapy with active assisted exercises and serial splinting can have significant benefits but treatment is time consuming. In resistant cases, where a flexion deformity of greater than 50° is present, then a surgical arthrolysis (Schindler et al, 1991; Amillo, 1992; Morrey, 1992; Boerboom et al, 1993) can be considered and may have a dramatic result. The results of arthrolysis have improved significantly with the perioperative use of continuous passive motion (CPM) machines (Boerboom et al, 1993). As the rheumatoid process progresses, three different problems develop:

- *Pain* – usually related to complete loss of articular cartilage from the joint, with bone articulating on bone.
- *Loss of movement* – most noticeably loss of full elbow extension (normally 0°), usually to fixed flexion of 40–70°; this is much less disabling than loss of full flexion (normally 140°), which commonly measures 90–120°.
- *Instability* of the elbow due to bone loss – the elbow starts to 'wobble' during normal activities and results in the patient feeling weakness of the arm and a tendency for the arm to give way under load.

Patients continue to be referred at a late stage of their disease for consideration for elbow arthroplasty. If excessive bone loss is present it can result in the elbow arthroplasty operation

Table 10.1 Larsen's classification of joints with rheumatoid arthritis

Grade 0	Normal conditions: abnormalities not related to arthritis (such as marginal bone deposition) may be present
Grade I	Slight abnormality. One or more of the following lesions are present: periarticular soft tissue swelling, periarticular osteoporosis and slight joint space narrowing. When possible comparison is made with a normal contralateral elbow or a previous radiograph of the joint in the same patient. The stage represents an early, uncertain phase of arthritis or a later phase without destruction
Grade II	Definite early abnormality. Erosion is obligatory except in the weight-bearing joints
Grade III	Medium destructive abnormality. Erosion and joint space narrowing corresponding to the standard radiographs. Erosion is obligatory in all joints
Grade IV	Severe destructive abnormality. Erosion and narrowing of the joint space. Bone deformation is present in the weight-bearing joints
Grade V	Mutilating abnormality. The original articular surfaces have disappeared. Gross bone deformation is present in the weight-bearing joints. Dislocation and bony ankylosis, being late and secondary, should not be considered in the grading; if present, the grading should be made according to the bone destruction or deformation

being a particularly difficult one because there may be insufficient bone stock for the fixation of the standard elbow replacement components. With improved medium term outcomes following total elbow replacement (TER) it is anticipated that earlier referrals will occur and this may be less of a problem in the future. For each surgeon the point at which elbow arthroplasty is offered depends on his or her personal experience, the stage of the disease and the severity of the patient's symptoms. Most surgeons will offer a TER to a rheumatoid patient when the pain is moderate or severe and the radiological changes are Larsen grade IV or V. Some patients with Larsen grade III changes will also be considered. The Larsen grading system (Larsen, Dale and Eek, 1977) has become established as the most practical and reproducible system and is summarized in Table 10.1.

However, the surgeon's decision to operate is not based only on the assessment of the elbow. The whole patient should be assessed because the treatment offered should result in a real benefit for the patient. With rheumatoid patients there is almost always other joint involvement in addition to the elbows; often the hands and wrists are badly affected by the rheumatoid process. It is illogical to improve elbow function if the hand is so crippled that the patient can gain little overall functional benefit from a TER. This assessment of the patient can be considerably aided by the occupational therapist and physiotherapist and it is common practice in some orthopaedic units for the patient to be referred for a full functional assessment by a therapist before being offered elbow replacement surgery. Having completed the evaluation of the patient it may be more appropriate to develop a complete treatment plan rather than just giving consideration to an elbow replacement. Firstly, 'Is the elbow the most painful joint?' If 'Yes', a TER might be justified. If 'No', would it be more appropriate to treat the most painful joint first – the shoulder or the lower limb joints for instance? In certain situations both the shoulder and the elbow may be replaced under the same general anaesthetic – simultaneous shoulder and elbow replacements. In our unit this has been used on over 15 occasions with very considerable patient satisfaction (Kocialkowski and Wallace, 1990; Neumann et al, 1994), but it is hard work for both the patient and the therapists.

Having made the decision to offer a TER there is some merit in entering the patient on to a waiting list, ideally delaying surgery for 3–6 months. Rheumatoid patients often fluctuate considerably in their symptomatology and by waiting a while the patient and surgeon can both be sure that the operation is truly justified. The British National Health Service normally ensures this delay is present but in other countries there may be a tendency to proceed straight to surgery with a little too much haste.

Other inflammatory arthritides with joint stiffness

The elbow is also affected by non-rheumatoid inflammatory arthritides such as psoriatic arthritis and ankylosing spondylitis. These conditions tend to cause elbow stiffness with joint space narrowing. Although they go through a painful stage during the acute inflammatory process, they tend to become pain free but stiff later. The management of such an elbow, which still has good bone stock and some joint space, is difficult. If the stiffness is severe then an arthrolysis operation with CPM would be appropriate. In some rare cases elbow arthroplasty might be appropriate but these patients tend to stress their joint replacements more than the rheumatoid patients and caution should be exercised in deciding to proceed to TER, as is discussed further in the section on post-traumatic osteoarthritis.

Osteoarthritis

There is considerable debate about the use of elbow arthroplasty for patients with primary osteoarthritis of the elbow. Many of these patients have carried out heavy manual work for many years (Stanley, 1993). They usually seek treatment because of loss of movement and pain on moving the elbow and they often wish to return to manual work. The strain such patients place on an elbow arthroplasty is very considerable and early and medium term loosening have been reported commonly in the past (Morrey, Adams and Bryan, 1991). There is general agreement at present that elbow arthroplasty is contraindicated 'for primary osteoarthritis except for patients who make low demands on the upper extremity or in elderly patients whose functional needs are similar to those of patients who have rheumatoid arthritis' (Ewald et al, 1993). Morrey (1992) and Redden and Stanley (1993) have shown that such patients can receive considerable benefit from an arthrolysis and debridement operation with postoperative CPM. This is therefore the first-line management of such a patient. Only in rare cases should TER be considered for primary osteoarthritis of the elbow. In such cases the patient should always be counselled about the need to avoid manual work after joint replacement in order to protect the joint from loosening.

Post-traumatic elbow stiffness with no deformity or arthritis

Some patients who have sustained an elbow injury develop marked elbow stiffness. This is most commonly seen as a result of inappropriate prolonged splintage of the elbow rather than as a direct consequence of the elbow injury itself. Radiographs of the elbow are required to check that no fractures are present and to exclude periarticular calcification – particularly myositis ossificans. If the radiographs are

normal with a good joint space present then there is *no* indication for arthroplasty. The operation of choice is a surgical arthrolysis with CPM, as discussed earlier.

Post-fracture elbow stiffness with deformity

Trauma is a frequent cause of elbow disability. Only since the mid-1980s has it become appreciated that for most displaced elbow fractures open reduction and internal fixation is the treatment of choice. Traditionally in Britain severe distal humeral fractures have been treated with the 'bag of bones' method with no operative intervention and early mobilization. Although these patients have a better result than the elbow which is simply immobilized, the outcomes are rarely good and frequently patients are left with elbow pain and deformity. In the 1990s even the severe distal humeral fractures are being considered for open reduction and internal fixation, with excellent results reported by Holdsworth and Mossad (1990) and Jupiter (1995). However, we have an ongoing group of patients who have unsatisfactory results after previous elbow fractures. These patients need to be carefully assessed by an orthopaedic surgeon with a special interest in the elbow. A number of cases can be improved dramatically with open surgery, corrective osteotomy and internal fixation. Experts have reported excellent results (Jupiter, 1995), but these results depend on careful preoperative planning of surgery and a surgeon with significant experience and expertise in this form of reconstructive surgery. Patients who have established non-union of complex distal humeral fractures are best treated with elbow capsulectomy, triple plating and ulnar nerve neurolysis (Jupiter and Goodman, 1992). Where the articular cartilage is in good condition and a good joint space can be demonstrated it is inappropriate to consider joint replacement. However, if the joint surfaces are extensively damaged then consideration should be given to joint replacement, as has been demonstrated by Figgie et al (1989a).

Post-traumatic osteoarthritis

Patients who have previously sustained a displaced elbow fracture may develop post-traumatic arthritis because of joint incongruity. It is remarkable how few seek an orthopaedic opinion when this happens – the majority seem to have only modest symptoms of elbow stiffness and some aching. There is a small group, however, who develop significant pain and are disabled by their arthritis and joint stiffness. These patients tend to be different from those with primary osteoarthritis; they are less likely to be involved in heavy manual work and they often make few demands on their elbows. These patients may be considered for TER after they have been counselled about the expected results from elbow arthroplasty but prosthetic surgery should be restricted to patients over 60 years (Morrey, Adams and Bryan, 1991). The operation will, however, be much more difficult than, for instance, an elbow arthroplasty for rheumatoid arthritis. The bone can be very sclerotic and hard to contour for the insertion of the prosthesis. The ligament attachments may be in the wrong place because of malunion of the bony fragments. The surgeon should ensure he or she is proficient in elbow arthroplasty for the rheumatoid patient before embarking on this form of difficult reconstructive surgery incorporating an arthroplasty.

Complete ankylosis of the elbow

Although elbow ankylosis is now rare there remain a few patients for whom arthroplasty may be appropriate. Complete ankylosis of the elbow can cause severe disability and functional limitations, especially when other joints in the ipsilateral upper extremity also have limited motion. Whilst complete ankylosis of the elbow usually results in diminished function, pain is seldom a problem. However, since pronation and supination are independent of flexion and extension, pain may be present due to disease of the radial head. Although the author has experience of only two cases of conversion of an elbow ankylosis to an arthroplasty, Figgie et al (1989b) have reported on 19 cases, 15 having a good or excellent result, and the reader is referred to their report for further information.

Preoperative assessment of the patient and consent for surgery

Before proceeding to arthroplasty the patient must be assessed for fitness for surgery. Rheumatoid arthritis patients are particular

surgical risks because of their multisystem disorder. Although it has become popular to treat such patients with antimitotic agents, the surgeon needs to be aware of the increased risk of sepsis which exists for patients on this medication, with deep infection rates of over 10% reported in such cases. These drugs should therefore be discontinued if possible 3 months before joint replacement surgery if possible. Particular care should focus on the cervical spine, where a lateral radiograph in flexion and extension should be obtained before general anaesthetic. The affected elbow should be examined for skin lesions (particularly infections) and to check the skin quality over the elbow. An up-to-date radiograph of the elbow should be available to ensure the anatomy is clearly displayed before surgery and, finally, ulnar nerve function should be checked clinically before surgery. A number of rheumatoid patients already have a mild ulnar neuritis as a consequence of their joint deformities and, if this is not identified before operation, the operation might be wrongly incriminated when the ulnar nerve function is assessed postoperatively.

Informed consent has become extremely important in relation to all surgical operations but particularly in the field of orthopaedic surgery. Patients should always be advised of the risks of surgery, and for elbow replacement these risks are considerable. The published results of the capitellocondylar, the Souter–Strathclyde and the Kudo elbow have been reviewed (Hodgson, Parkinson and Noble, 1991; Poll and Rozing, 1991; Ruth and Wilde, 1992; Souter, 1992; Ewald et al, 1993). The following are the risks, together with their estimated frequency, which the patients will undergo if they proceed to a total elbow arthroplasty:

- General risks: Myocardial infarction (MI) = 1–3%
  Death from MI = 1%
  Pulmonary embolism (PE) = 3–5%
  Death from PE = 1%
- Local risks: Transient ulnar nerve damage = up to 65%
  Permanent ulnar nerve damage = up to 10%
  Deep infection = 0–8%
  Long-term instability (dislocation) = 4–10%
  Aseptic loosening = up to 10% at 10 years

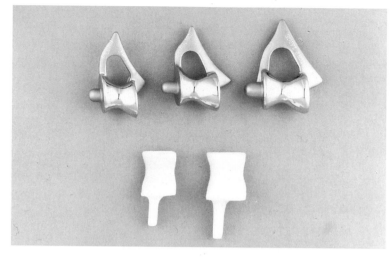

(a)

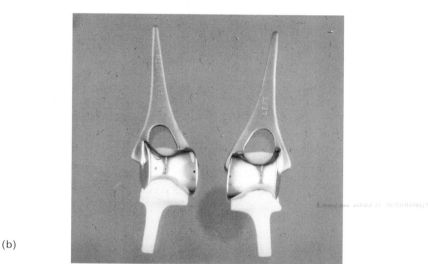

(b)

Figure 10.1 (a) and (b) Souter–Strathclyde total elbow replacement.

For rheumatoid arthritis the prosthesis survival rate at an average of 5 years is between 83 and 90% for the capitellocondylar (Ruth and Wilde 1992; Ewald et al, 1993), between 89 and 95% for the Souter–Strathclyde (Poll and Rozing, 1991; Souter, 1992) and 89% for the Kudo (Kudo and Iwano, 1990). For post-traumatic osteoarthritis the revision rate using the Coonrad TER has been reported to be 18% at an average follow-up period of 6.3 years (Morrey, Adams and Bryan, 1991).

Prostheses for total elbow replacement

Different surgeons use different prostheses for TER. They select their favoured prosthesis for a number of reasons: it was the prosthesis which they learned to use first; it was the prosthesis their hospital used; one of their colleagues recommended it; etc. Since the beginning of the 1990s, however, it has become possible to select the prosthesis more scientifically using the results reported from follow-up studies. On the basis of these recent reports, three particular prostheses have emerged as the current most popular and successful prostheses in Europe: the capitellocondylar, the Souter–Strathclyde and the Kudo Type 4 TERs. These will therefore be described in more detail, although mention will be made of the more constrained prostheses which may be used in special circumstances.

Capitellocondylar TER

This prosthesis (see Figure 8.4) was developed in Boston, Massachusetts by Ewald and was introduced for clinical use in 1974. It was introduced when the problems of constrained elbow hinges began to emerge and the capitello-condylar was one of the first non-constrained prostheses to be used clinically. The results in clinical use have now been reported by Ewald et al (1993) in 202 cases, Weiland et al (1989) in 40 cases, Ruth and Wilde (1992) in 51 cases and Hodgson, Parkinson and Noble (1991) in 23 cases. This prosthesis is marketed in the UK by Johnson & Johnson Orthopaedics.

Souter–Strathclyde TER

Having reviewed the relatively poor results of early elbow arthroplasties (Souter, 1973), Souter from Edinburgh, in collaboration with Nicol, Paul and Berme at the Bioengineering Unit of the University of Strathclyde, developed a stirrup-shaped humeral prosthesis which improved the anchorage of the component by fully utilizing the contours of the medullary cavities of the medial and lateral supracondylar ridges (Souter, Nicol and Paul, 1985). The design is shown in Figure 10.1. The initial prosthesis was developed with an all poly-ethylene ulnar component; it came into clinical use in 1977 and in the UK is marketed by Howmedica International. Clinical reports on the results using the Souter–Strathclyde TER have been published by Poll and Rozing (1991) in 34 cases, Souter (1992) in 136 cases and Zafiropoulos and Lunn (Zafiropoulos, 1994) in 48 cases. In cases where the distal humeral bone is deficient, or has fractured peroperatively, the long-stemmed 'revision' humeral component is recommended.

Kudo Type 4 TER

Kudo from Sagamihara Hospital, Japan developed his own surface replacement with no stem on the humeral component – the Type 1. This was used clinically from 1971 to 1975. The humeral component was modified to incorporate a saddle shape with a trochlea in the centre, more like the natural articulation – the Type 2; this was used from 1975 until 1983. Because of sinkage of some of the humeral components a stem was added for use with cement in 1983 –

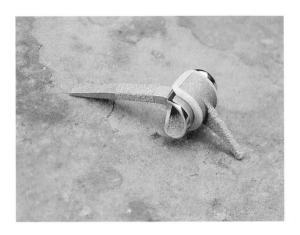

Figure 10.2 Kudo (Type 4) total elbow replacement. (Courtesy of Biomet Ltd.)

the Type 3. The Type 4 prosthesis with a porous coated stem to promote biological fixation was introduced in 1988 and is the design currently marketed by Biomet Ltd (Figure 10.2). Early clinical results for the Type 1 and Type 2 were reported in 1980 in 24 cases (Kudo, Iwano and Watanabe, 1980) and long-term results for the Type 1 and Type 2 in 1990 in 37 cases (Kudo and Iwano, 1990). The results for the Type 4 Kudo have only been presented orally but one report has highlighted stem breakage in eight of the 34 prototype Type 4 humeral components inserted (H. Kudo, personal communication 1994). The manufacturers have now strengthened the stem and stem breakage is now rare.

Pooley from Newcastle-upon-Tyne in England is co-ordinating the clinical trials of this prosthesis (J. Pooley, personal communication 1994). To date, 2500 prostheses have been inserted, with very positive feedback about how much easier this prosthesis is to insert than other TERs.

Coonrad–Morrey TER

This prosthesis is a semiconstrained device. It was initially designed in 1969 and developed and marketed in 1970. In 1978 the design was modified to the Coonrad II to permit 7° of hinge laxity or toggle in order to reduce bone–cement interface forces. In 1981 the prosthesis was further modified by the Mayo Clinic to the current design – the Coonrad–Morrey with a band of porous coating of the distal humerus and proximal ulnar stems to promote biological

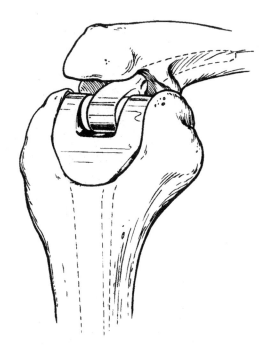

Figure 10.3 Coonrad–Morrey total elbow replacement.

fixation, although the marketing company (Zimmer Inc.) state: 'This implant is intended to be used with bone cement for immediate and long-term fixation. There are no known indications for implanting this device without cement'!! (Coonrad and Morrey, 1989). Clinical results have been reported by Morrey et al in 55 cases (of post-traumatic arthritis) (Morrey, Adams and Bryan, 1991).

Pritchard Mark II floppy hinged prosthesis

This prosthesis has generally been restricted for use only in difficult clinical cases with bone loss and damage to soft tissues. The prosthesis was originally designed by Pritchard and Walker (Pritchard, 1981). Late complications of wear and loosening have now been reported (Madsen, Sojbjerg and Sneppen, 1994) and the author does not recommend its use.

Link prosthesis

This prosthesis is reserved for cases which have massive bone loss in the elbow region and loss of the stabilizing soft tissues necessary for a surface replacement design. It has only been used in a limited number of cases but has been found to be a valuable salvage prosthesis in

Denmark and Nottingham. An illustration of the prosthesis, which incorporates stems for humerus, radius and ulna, is shown in Figure 10.3. Long-term results are not available for this cementless design of prosthesis.

Surgical techniques for total elbow replacement

Positioning of patient and tourniquet

The patient is positioned in a semilateral position with the upper arm supported in a short arm support, as shown in Figure 10.5. A well-padded pneumatic tourniquet is applied high up the upper arm and inflated after partial exsanguination of the arm by simple elevation. It is important to check that the elbow can be comfortably flexed to over 110° when in this position to facilitate access to the elbow during surgery.

Surgical approach

There are a number of surgical approaches that can be used for elbow arthroplasty. These include the Campbell posterior approach (Campbell, 1932), a modified Kocher approach (Ewald and Jacobs, 1984), an extensive posterior exposure (Bryan and Morrey, 1982) or the osteoanconeus flap (Wolfe and Ranawat, 1990). The author's preferred approach, a modified posterior Campbell approach, has been influenced by the reported frequency of ulnar nerve symptoms after elbow arthroplasty, with figures as high as 65% for temporary nerve dysfunction reported using the Kocher approach (Hodgson, Parkinson and Noble, 1991). A straight posterior midline incision about 20 cm long through skin and subcutaneous fat is carried down to the triceps aponeurosis (Figure 10.5). The skin flaps are then reflected as far as the medial and lateral epicondyles. The ulnar nerve should now be dissected free from its bed in the cubital fossa and mobilized for a maximum distance of 4 cm above and below the elbow. Particular care should be taken to free the nerve as it passes distally between the two heads of the flexor carpi ulnaris muscle, and any ligamentous band crossing over it should be divided. A moist tape or Penrose drain may be used with care as a sling to gently retract the nerve to protect it during the operation (Figure

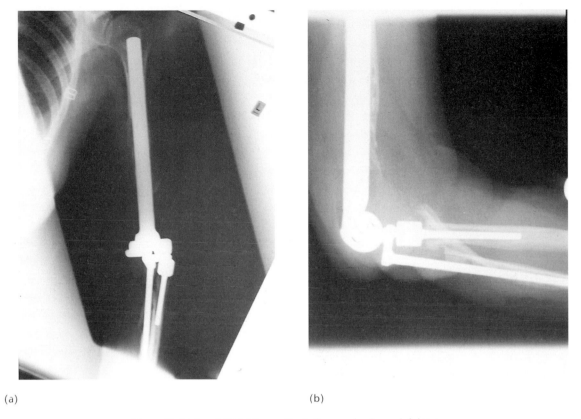

(a)

(b)

Figure 10.4 (a) and (b) Link prosthesis for massive bone deficiency.

10.6). An 8 cm long U-shaped posterior triceps aponeurosis flap is now created, with mobilization of the triceps tendon from its proximal muscle attachment. The aponeurosis is dissected off the underlying long and medial heads of the triceps muscle using sharp dissection (Figure 10.7). The lateral incision is extended distally along the lateral border of the proximal ulna and the anconeus muscle is separated from its attachment to the ulna. The incision is deepened in the region of the olecranon fosssa and the annular ligament is separated from its origin and tagged with a stay suture. The triceps flap is reflected distally and downwards, wrapped in a moist swab and tacked on to the underlying deep fascia (Figure 10.8). The posterior capsule of the elbow is divided with a midline incision and detached from the olecranon (Figure 10.9). Retraction on the annular ligament with some further release of soft tissues from the ulna now allows access to the radial head and neck. Dissection should not be carried too far distally because of the risk of injury to the posterior interosseous nerve. The radial neck can now be visualized and osteotomized, preferably with an oscillating saw, to allow excision of the radial head (Figure 10.10). A partial synovectomy may be performed if the synovium is hypertrophic. To facilitate dislocation of the elbow, all adhesions between the joint surfaces should now be cleared. There is controversy about the surgical management of the medial collateral ligament. For both the capitellocondylar (Ewald et al, 1993) and the Souter–Strathclyde (Souter, 1983) it has been recommended that the medial collateral ligament should be preserved, while for the Kudo (Kudo and Iwano, 1990) it is recommended that the medial collateral ligament including the tight anterior bundle should be released. However, the author agrees with the observation of Pooley (J. Pooley, personal communication 1994) that the medial olecranon osteophyte, which is almost always present in rheumatoid patients and can be very large, often replaces the medial collateral ligament. If the osteophyte is excised the ligament is often defunctioned. It has become the author's policy to divide the

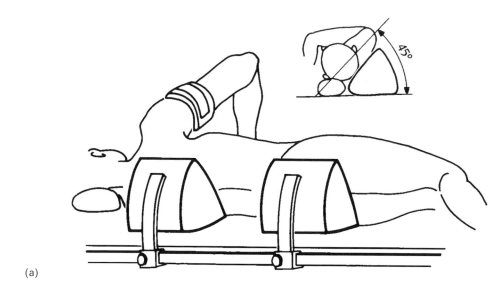

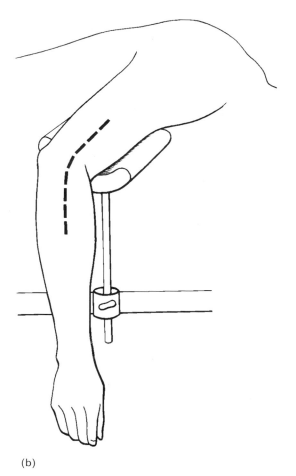

(b)

Figure 10.5 Patient positioning for total elbow replacement

ligament electively, as described by Kudo (Kudo and Iwano, 1990). Gentle retraction on the ulnar nerve at this stage of the operation protects it from injury. The whole of the elbow is now exposed for preparation of the bone for the selected prosthesis. The exact technique for each of the elbow arthroplasties is described clearly in the manufacturer's brochures and videotapes but comments on the particular points of emphasis and the technical difficulties are summarized in the following sections.

Capitellocondylar prosthesis

Ewald has recommended that this is put in through a Kocher approach in order to protect the ulnar nerve, but experience in both Britain and the USA has highlighted that the problem of short-term ulnar neuritis (65% in Britain and 15 or 16% in the USA) and long-term ulnar nerve palsy (4% in Britain and 5 or 3% in the USA) still remain (Weiland et al, 1989; Hodgson, Parkinson and Noble, 1991; Ewald et al, 1993). Weiland, who has extensive experience of the capitellocondylar prosthesis, has stated that: 'The surgical technique for the placement of an unconstrained total elbow prosthesis is challenging, and more attention to the quality and repair of the soft tissues is needed than with the constrained designs.' (Weiland et al, 1989).

The incidence of aseptic loosening in the capitellocondylar prosthesis is low, with 0/40 cases of loosening reported by Weiland (Weiland et al, 1989), 3/202 cases reported by Ewald

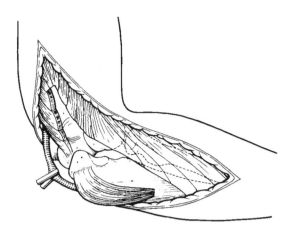

Figure 10.8 U-shaped posterior triceps flap.

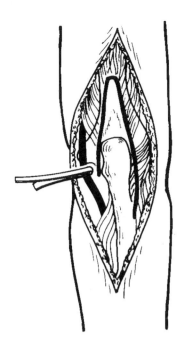

Figure 10.6 The skin incision.

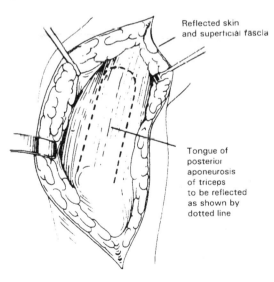

Reflected skin and superficial fascia

Tongue of posterior aponeurosis of triceps to be reflected as shown by dotted line

Figure 10.7 Mobilization and gentle retraction of the ulnar nerve.

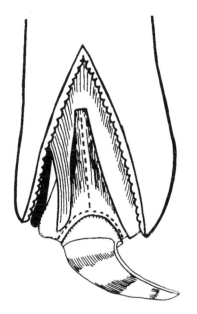

Figure 10.9 The posterior elbow capsule is opened through a midline incision with a distal T extension.

(Ewald et al, 1993). However, the incidence of dislocation is high: 3.5% (Ewald et al, 1993); 5% (Weiland et al, 1989). This is in part thought to relate to ensuring the components are aligned correctly (with the humeral component placed 5° internally rotated with respect to the transepicondylar line), as well as to the meticulous reconstruction of the soft tissues.

Souter–Strathclyde TER

This prosthesis is currently used extensively in the UK and in Europe. The recommended surgical approach is the posterior Campbell, and the incidence of temporary ulnar nerve symptoms was found to be 15% (Souter, 1992) and of permanent ulnar nerve palsy 6% (Poll and Rozling, 1991; Zafiropoulos, 1994). All surgeons using this prosthesis have found it a challenging surgical technique with serious risks

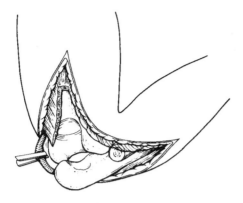

Figure 10.10 Extension of the incision along the lateral side of the ulna. The radial neck is asteotomized and the elbow is fully exposed, ready for preparation of the bone cuts.

of peroperative complications, particularly fracture of the epicondyles or the olecranon, around the time of completion of bone preparation. Souter has reported no aseptic loosening in 131 TERs but 5 loosenings did occur secondary to epicondylar and olecranon fractures (Souter, 1992). Poll has reported aseptic loosening in 4/34 TERs (Poll and Rozing, 1991), while Zafiropoulos and Lunn have warned that, although they had no clinical loosening, 43% of elbows had a radiolucent line of at least 2 cm around part of the ulnar component (Zafiropoulos, 1994). Dislocation has been a problem with this prosthesis, with rates of 3% (Souter, 1992), 5% (Zafiropoulos, 1994) and 9% (Poll and Rozing, 1991) reported.

Kudo Type 4 TER

Again, ulnar nerve symptoms have occurred with the use of this prosthesis inserted through a posterior Campbell approach. In 4/37 (11%) patients an early ulnar nerve palsy occurred, with 2/37 (5%) having permanent symptoms (Kudo and Iwano, 1990). The results with regard to loosening are difficult to analyse because Kudo has reported the long-term results of his two early designs (Types 1 and 2) (Kudo and Iwano, 1990), while the currently used prosthesis (the Type 4) has only a short postoperative follow-up. The Type 1 and Type 2 have a reported dislocation rate of 5% (Kudo and Iwano, 1990). The type 4 prosthesis has been found particularly attractive to surgeons because, by comparison with the capitello-

condylar and Souter–Strathclyde, it is much easier to insert. Unfortunately, this advantage must be balanced against a recently reported 8/34 (24%) breakage rate for the stem of the prototype Type 4 humeral component (H. Kudo, personal communication 1994). Pooley from Newcastle, who is co-ordinating the clinical trials of the Kudo elbow, has confirmed that over 2500 Type 4 Kudo elbows have been inserted and feels that Professor Kudo's surgical technique and the use of prototype (titanium alloy) implants might be the cause of stem fracture (J. Pooley, personal communication 1994). Gallacher from Norwich, England has inserted 120 Type 4 Kudo elbows since 1991 with no stem breakages (Gallacher, 1994).

Drainage and closure

For all non-constrained elbow arthroplasty designs the reconstruction of the soft tissues when closing the wound is emphasized. Although there is controversy about the need to preserve the medial collateral ligament, there is universal agreement that the lateral collateral ligament should be carefully reconstructed during the closure. This is most conveniently carried out by firmly reattaching the divided origin of the annular ligament (to which the lateral collateral ligament is attached) to the lateral side of the ulna with strong non-absorbable sutures, e.g. no. 2 Ethibond (Ethicon). The author recommends that the tourniquet should be deflated at this stage, which allows good haemostasis to be obtained before skin closure. Next, the ulnar nerve is checked to ensure it has not been damaged during the operation or deep closure. The author recommends that the nerve should be returned to its groove behind the medial epicondyle and retained there with one loosely applied absorbable (Vicryl) suture which does not constrict the nerve in any way. To date anterior transposition has not been proven to be necessary. Two Redivac (Biomet) vacuum drains are now inserted and meticulous two-layer skin closure is effected with either subcuticular sutures to skin or skin clips.

Postoperative dressings

A non-adherent wound dressing is recommended, held on with a gently but firmly applied wool and crepe bandage while the elbow is held at 90° flexion. The author does not use any backslab or cast immobilization.

Postoperative mobilization programme

At 48 hours the dressings are reduced and early active and assisted flexion–extension and pronation–supination movements are started. If available, a CPM machine is used for up to four periods of 2–4 hours each during the day. The skin on the point of the elbow is particularly vulnerable to pressure sores and the routine use of a sheepskin elbow protector in the postoperative period, and perhaps even in the long term for patients with very fragile skin, is recommended. The postoperative rehabilitation is of great importance to the final range of motion and is fully covered in Chapter 12.

Surgical complications and their management

Postoperative complications after TER are common. They can be divided into (1) complications from the surgical exposure, and (2) complications directly related to the prosthesis.

Complications from the surgical exposure

The skin around the elbow is thin with often only a thin layer of subcutaneous fat. Care should be taken when handling the skin edges during the operation and direct undermining of the skin should be avoided – the plane of dissection is between the subcutaneous fat and the triceps aponeurosis. Good haemostasis should be carried out and this is facilitated by an incomplete exsanguination at the start of the operation, allowing better visualization of the blood vessels. Vacuum drainage is strongly recommended, with firm pressure bandaging at completion of the operation to reduce haematoma formation. A gentle suturing technique or the use of atraumatic skin clips should be used for the skin closure. The skin of the wound should be inspected at the time the wound is redressed at 48 hours to check all is well. Any problems such as haematoma or loss of skin viability should be tackled early, if necessary with the assistance of a plastic surgeon.

Ulnar nerve problems should be looked for at the time of the immediate postoperative check.

If a partial ulnar nerve lesion is found it should be observed for 10 days and, if no improvement occurs, exploration, decompression and possible superficial anterior transposition should be considered. It is the author's usual policy *not* to transpose the ulnar nerve. If a complete nerve lesion is identified in the postoperative period, then the nerve should be re-explored early to be sure that it has not been injured surgically by division or traumatized with an ensnaring suture.

Complications directly related to the prosthesis

Preoperative fractures should be avoided by careful handling of the bone. If these do occur the use of a longer-stemmed implant may be required and these should always be available at the start of every primary TER. Instability and dislocation of the unconstrained prostheses remain a real problem. Malposition of the implants has been particularly emphasized and is now thought to be the most common cause of dislocation (Souter, 1983; Briggs and Smith, 1993; Ewald et al, 1993). It is likely that further work will focus on helping the surgeon to improve the orientation of the implants. Management of dislocation has involved either accepting the dislocation and reviewing the patient as necessary or revision surgery. However, revision surgery is associated with a very significant risk of infection: 2 of 4 in Lunn's series (Zafiropoulos, 1994). Aseptic loosening will occur with all current implants and may become an increasing problem related to duration of implantation. Deep infection is fortunately uncommon. When it occurs, early surgical management is necessary. The author recommends initial removal of the whole prosthesis and all cement and the application of an external fixator to the midshaft of the humerus and ulna to provide initial stabilization. The wounds are allowed to heal and the surgeon will then decide on either revision elbow replacement or excision arthroplasty at 8 weeks after removal of the implant. The recent successful management of two such cases over a period of 8 years has confirmed this policy to be practical. Wolfe et al (1990) have reported their very considerable experience of the management of 14 cases of deep infection at the Hospital for Special Surgery in New York and the reader is referred to their paper for further advice.

Conclusions

Total elbow replacement has now become a standard orthopaedic operation. It is regularly used for rheumatoid arthritis and for some cases of post-traumatic arthritis. Most surgeons believe that the current prosthesis will develop mechanical loosening if used for younger, fit osteoarthritic patients, and alternative treatments are recommended for these patients. The surgeon has a responsibility to the patient to ensure at operation that the risks of infection are reduced to an absolute minimum and that particular care is taken to protect the radial nerve during surgery. One of the author's patients, who had an excellent result from her elbow arthroplasty but who sustained a significant ulnar nerve palsy, commented that she was pleased that she had had the operation because of the pain relief but her disability had now moved from the elbow to the hand!

The ideal prosthesis should provide reliable long-term results and should be capable of insertion by an orthopaedic surgeon with average skills. These aims have not yet been fully achieved but the prostheses being used in the 1990s are very much better than those in use in the 1960s. The main long-term concern is mechanical loosening and breakage of the prosthesis – problems which are likely to remain in the foreseeable future.

References

Amillo S (1991) Arthrolysis in the relief of post-traumatic stiffness of the elbow. *International Orthopaedics* **16** 188–190.

Boerboom AL, de Meyier HE, Berburg AD and Verhaar JAN (1993) Arthrolysis for post-traumatic stiffness of the elbow. *International Orthopaedics* **17** 346–349.

Briggs PJ and Smith SR (1993) Radiographic assessment of component orientation in elbow arthroplasty – a technical description. *Acta Orthopaedica Scandinavica* **64** 212–215.

Bryan RS and Morrey BF (1982) Extensive posterior exposure of the elbow: a triceps-sparing approach. *Clinical Orthopaedics and Related Research* **166** 188–192.

Campbell WC (1932) Incision for exposure of the elbow joint. *American Journal of Surgery* **15** 65–67.

Coonrad R W and Morrey B F (1989) *Coonrad/Morrey total elbow: surgical technique*. Zimmer Inc. Product Information.

Ewald FC and Jacobs MA (1984) Total elbow arthroplasty. *Clinical Orthopaedics and Related Research* **182** 137–142.

Ewald FC, Simmons ED, Sullivan JA et al (1993) Capitellocondylar total elbow replacement in rheumatoid arthritis – long-term results. *Journal of Bone and Joint Surgery* **75A** 498–507.

Figgie MP, Inglis AE, Mow CS and Figgie HE III (1989a) Salvage of non-union of supracondylar fracture of the humerus by total elbow arthroplasty. *Journal of Bone and Joint Surgery* **71A** 1058–1065.

Figgie MP, Inglis AE, Mow CS and Figgie HE III (1989b) Total elbow arthroplasty for complete ankylosis of the elbow. *Journal of Bone and Joint Surgery* **71A** 513–520.

Gallacher, P. Results from the Kudo Type 4 prosthesis. 1994.

Hodgson SP, Parkinson RW and Noble J (1991) Capitellocondylar total elbow replacement for rheumatoid arthritis. *Journal of the Royal College of Surgeons of Edinburgh* **36** 133–135.

Holdsworth BJ and Mossad MM (1990) Fractures of the distal humerus, elbow function after internal fixation. *Journal of Bone and Joint Surgery* **72B** 362–365.

Jupiter JB and Goodman LJ (1992) The management of complex distal humerus nonunion in the elderly by elbow capsulectomy, triple plating, and ulnar nerve neurolysis. *Journal of Shoulder and Elbow Surgery* **1** 37 46.

Jupiter JB (1995) Complex fracture of the distal part of the humerus and associated complications. *Instructional Course Lectures, American Academy of Orthopaedic Surgery* **44** 187–198.

Kocialkowski A and Wallace W A (1990) One-stage arthroplasty of the ipsilateral shoulder and elbow. *Journal of Bone and Joint Surgery* **72B** 520.

Kudo H and Iwano K (1990) Total elbow arthroplasty with a non-constrained surface-replacement prosthesis in patients who have rheumatoid arthritis: a long-term follow-up study. *Journal of Bone and Joint Surgery* **72A** 355–362.

Kudo H, Iwano K and Watanabe S (1980) Total replacement of the rheumatoid elbow with a hingeless prosthesis. *Journal of Bone and Joint Surgery* **62A** 277–285.

Larsen A, Dale K and Eek M (1977) Radiographic evaluation of rheumatoid arthritis and related conditions by standard reference films. *Acta Radiologica; Diagnosis* **18** 481–491.

Madsen F, Sojbjerg JO and Sneppen O (1994) Late complications with the Pritchard Mark II elbow prosthesis. *Journal of Shoulder and Elbow Surgery* **3** 17–23.

Morrey BF (1992) Primary degenerative arthritis of the elbow – treatment by ulnohumeral arthroplasty. *Journal of Bone and Joint Surgery* **74B** 409–413.

Morrey BF, Adams RA and Bryan RS (1991) Total replacement for post-traumatic arthritis of the elbow. *Journal of Bone and Joint Surgery* **73B** 607–612.

Neumann L, Frostick SP, Wallace WA, Damrel D and Mackie A (1994) Ipsilateral shoulder and elbow arthroplasty in the rheumatoid patient at one operating session. *Journal of Shoulder and Elbow Surgery* **3** S18.

Poll RG and Rozing PM (1991) Use of the Souter–Strathclyde total elbow prosthesis in patients who have rheumatoid arthritis. *Journal of Bone and Joint Surgery* **73A** 1227–1233.

Pritchard RW (1981) Long-term follow-up study: semi-constrained elbow prosthesis. *Orthopedics* **4** 151–155.

Redden JF and Stanley D (1993) Arthroscopic fenestration of the olecranon fossa in the treatment of osteoarthritis of the elbow. *Arthroscopy* **9**(1) 14–16.

Ruth, JT and Wilde AH (1992) Capitellocondylar total elbow replacement. *Journal of Bone and Joint Surgery* **74A** 95–100.

Schindler A, Yaffe B, Chetrit A et al. (1991) Factors influencing elbow arthrolysis. *Annales de Chirurgie de la Main et du Membre Superieure* **10** 237–242.

Souter WA (1973) Arthroplasty of the elbow – with particular reference to metallic hinge arthroplasty in rheumatoid patients. *Orthopedic Clinics of North America* **4** 395–413.

Souter WA (1983) *Howmedica surgical techniques: Souter–Strathclyde arthroplasty of elbow.* London: Howmedica.

Souter WA (1992) Souter–Strathclyde arthroplasty in the management of the adult rheumatoid elbow – results at five and ten year follow-up. *Proceedings of the Ninth Combined Meeting of the Orthopaedic Associations of the English-Speaking World* (1992): Paper 76.

Souter WA, Nicol AC and Paul JP (1985) Anatomical trochlea stirrup arthroplasty of the rheumatoid elbow. *Journal of Bone and Joint Surgery* **67B** 676.

Stanley D (1993) The prevalence and aetiological aspects of primary osteoarthritis of the elbow. *Journal of Bone and Joint Surgery* **75B** (Suppl.) 41.

Weiland AJ, Weiss A-PC, Wills RP and Moore JR (1989) Capitellocondylar total elbow replacement. *Journal of Bone and Joint Surgery* **71A** 217–222.

Wolfe SW and Ranawat CS (1990) The osteo-anconeus flap – an approach for total elbow arthroplasty. *Journal of Bone and Joint Surgery* **72A** 684–688.

Wolfe SW, Figgie MP, Inglis AE, Bohn WH and Ranawat CS (1990) Management of infection about total elbow prostheses. *Journal of Bone and Joint Surgery* **73A** 198 212.

Zafiropoulos G (1994) Total elbow replacement: Biomechanics and outcome. MPhil Thesis, University of Nottingham, 1994.

11

Revision elbow arthroplasty

John K. Stanley and Peter G. Lunn

The development of joint replacement surgery has brought with it the realization that the salvage potential of the arthroplasty is almost as important as the basic design itself. In the event of failure of the arthroplasty in the future, there must be some means of allowing the patient to preserve some useful function. The aim of joint replacement is to relieve pain and restore or maintain stability and movement, and hence function. An operation to achieve this excellent ideal must not risk the loss of all function and the return of pain and instability, otherwise one of the basic reasons for the procedure has not been realized. This is of particular importance in the elbow as the salvage procedures are limited. One of the main criticisms of some of the earlier designs of elbow arthroplasty, particularly the early 'hinges', was that they involved much resection of bone and later were often associated with further resorption of bone due to subsequent loosening, such that salvage procedures were virtually impossible. The only option if the arthroplasty failed was to leave the patient with an unstable, flail elbow.

The salvage options following failed primary elbow replacement include revision to another arthroplasty – of the same or a different design, excision arthroplasty, arthrodesis, allograft implantation, or finally amputation. These techniques may have to be considered but all have their own shortcomings which will be discussed.

It is well known, but worth emphasizing, that in the present 'state of the art' the primary arthroplasty is the best chance of achieving a good result and both the patient and the surgeon must accept that any salvage procedure can only be expected to have limited success, both in terms of relief of symptoms and return of function. It is hoped that the discussion of the causes of failure and their treatment may give an insight to the primary surgeon who will better understand the pitfalls associated with total elbow replacement and perhaps by so doing will reduce the need for revision surgery.

This chapter will deal mainly with revision from one arthroplasty to another, either of the same or a different type. First, however, we will discuss some of the reasons for failure of the primary arthroplasty, then look in more detail at the salvage procedures available and some of the techniques and equipment required to undertake this type of surgery.

Causes of failure

The range of elbow implants used over the years has included: simple shell resurfacing replacements with virtually no fixation; linked, fully constrained hinges; 'sloppy' constrained hinges; semiconstrained anatomical total joint replacement; and unconstrained implants. This variety of implants and the variations within each type would suggest a wide range of reasons for failure, but it is possible to group these causes into one or other of the following five main categories:

1 Chronic instability (with or without pain).
2 Implant loosening (with or without fracture).
3 Implant failure.
4 Infection.
5 Patient selection factors.

A poor range of movement after prosthetic replacement of the elbow is rarely an indication for revision unless it is associated with some other problem such as implant loosening or failure, or if there was some technical error made during the original procedure.

Chronic instability

The stability of the normal elbow joint is maintained by a combination of the bony structure and the soft tissues. Frequently the bony configuration has been altered or replaced to a greater or lesser extent by the primary arthroplasty and may provide some inherent stability; but most arthroplasties rely heavily on the soft tissue support and if this is deficient then they tend to sublux or dislocate, as is seen in Figure 11.1 where a Wadsworth Mark 1 elbow has subluxed because of failure of the medial collateral ligament.

The main structures providing soft tissue support after elbow arthroplasty are:

1 the medial collateral ligament – particularly the anterior portion
2 the lateral collateral ligament – including the annular ligament
3 the anconeus muscle
4 the triceps insertion
5 the brachialis muscle and anterior capsule inserted into the coronoid process.

Deficiencies in any of these soft tissue stabilizers can lead to different types of instability. Loss of the anterior structures with attenuation of the collateral ligaments allows pure posterior subluxation or full dislocation. Loss of the triceps expansion and the anconeus muscle results in posteromedial and supination instability, whereas failure of the medial structures gives rise to cubitus valgus deformity, often with considerable pain, and sometimes associated with a tardy ulnar palsy.

Revision for instability demands that the underlying soft tissue failure is repaired or replaced in some way before the joint replace-

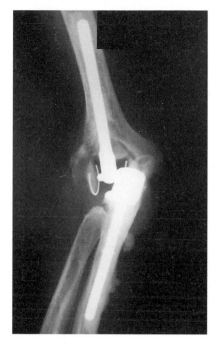

Figure 11.1 Radiograph of a long-stemmed Wadsworth Mark 3 elbow replacement. The medial ligament has failed and the components are subluxing.

ment is revised. Sometimes this is not difficult; at other times it may be impossible and so the stability of the joint may have to be achieved in some other way.

Failure of the triceps tendon and attenuation of the anconeus muscle can be readily repaired by careful dissection of the two layers followed by a two-layer closure; the anconeus is attached to the ulna at the edge of the olecranon and the triceps tendon is either repaired directly or reconstructed with strips of fascia lata or proximal triceps tendon.

Repair of the medial collateral ligament is very much more difficult, not only because of the proximity of the ulnar nerve, which must be mobilized to allow sufficient access, but also because the isometric line of the medial ligament must be assessed accurately so that the reconstructed ligament can be positioned correctly; failure to do so will either result in persisting instability or else restriction of elbow movement, or at worst, both. The isometric line, shown in Figure 11.2, is usually closely related to the anterior portion of the medial ligament and this ligament can be reconstructed by taking a palmaris longus or fascia lata graft and attaching this on the medial side to the medial epicondyle and laterally to the medial

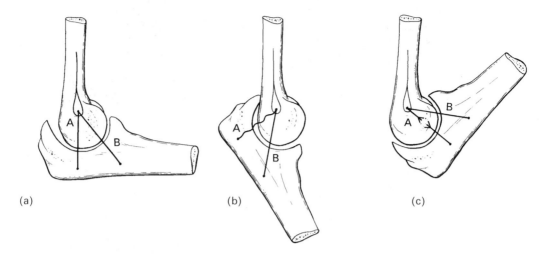

(a)   (b)   (c)

Figure 11.2 (a)–(c) A is the longitudinal axis of the humerus; B is the isometric line which is the line of attachment of the anterior portion of the medial ligament and is the correct position for any medial ligament reconstruction.

aspect of the olecranon or to the coronoid process in the region of the coronoid tubercle. This type of ligamentous reconstruction requires postoperative protection for 3 months in a hinged splint allowing a restricted range of flexion and extension in order to prevent excessive stresses on the ligament.

Chronic posterior instability is also a difficult problem to solve. Reattachment of the anterior structures to the coronoid has been disappointing in our very limited experience and we recommend tight repair of the medial and lateral structures (which is more readily achieved from a posterior approach) followed by postoperative protection in an extension-block splint for 3 months. Restriction of full extension by 30–40° allows the anterior capsule and brachialis muscle to heal tightly and will prevent further posterior instability. Fortunately this restriction of movement rarely causes any serious functional disability.

Implant loosening

Loosening of an implant is usually a slow process which can only be confirmed after extensive long-term follow-up. However, chronic progressive loosening of an arthroplasty, especially some of the early elbow hinges, can be associated with extensive bony erosion and resorption, sometimes culminating in pathological fracture. Any form of functional salvage procedure is virtually impossible in this situation and hopefully nowadays the signs of loosening can be recognized at an early stage and treatment instituted before this scenario has developed.

In the authors' personal series of elbow arthroplasties it is interesting to note that, even in a relatively short follow-up period of up to 6 years, there are features of our surgical technique which we have had to modify because of the 'risk factors' seen at review, even though the clinical results have been largely satisfactory.

A 3–6-year review of an anatomical, semi-constrained implant (the Souter–Strathclyde arthroplasty) has shown that in 50 patients at one centre (Wrightington) there were three features which could be highlighted as high-risk factors with regard to the possibility of future loosening of the humeral components.

1 *The size of the humeral component* If the humeral component is not sufficiently large there will not be adequate fixation of the shoulders of the component into the supracondylar ridges. It is therefore important to use the largest humeral component that can be accommodated comfortably.

2 *The medial supracondylar ridge* If the humeral component is positioned too far medially this will weaken the medial supracondylar ridge and may lead to fracture at the time of operation or loosening at a later stage (Figure 11.4). This

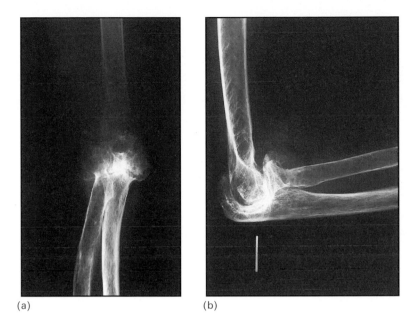

(a)   (b)

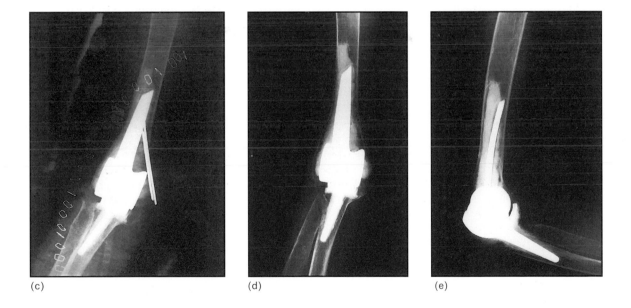

(c)   (d)   (e)

Figure 11.3 Loosening of the humeral component. Preoperative radiographs; (a) AP and (b) Lateral views. Postoperative radiograph: (c) AP – Wadsworth Mark 2 showing fracture of the medial epicondyle which was fixed with two K-wires. Follow-up radiographs: (d) AP and (e) lateral views showing radiological signs of loosening. 'Cement lines' seen at the interface between the humeral component and the cement and also at the bone–cement interface.

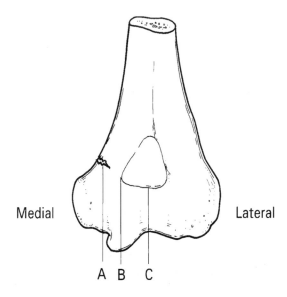

Medial   Lateral

A B C

Figure 11.4 Alignment of the medial edge of the humeral component is critical to the long-term result: line A is too medial – high risk of fracture of the medial ridge; line B is correct – supracondylar ridge intact; line C is too lateral – implant will be too small, medial fixation may be inadequate resulting in more risk of loosening.

medial placement can occur either as a result of malalignment or because the humeral component is too large and necessitates excessive excavation of the medial epicondyle and supracondylar ridge. Fractures occurred in three patients in this series and, although the wiring and cementing appear to allow the fractures to unite, all three cases have progressed to either radiological or frank clinical loosening (Figure 11.3).

3 *Rotation of the humeral component* When seen from the lateral view the humeral component should be in line with the longitudinal axis of the humerus. In the longer-stemmed prostheses this is less of a problem, although it does occur, but in the Souter–Strathclyde arthroplasty the shorter stem can be rotated so that the superior tip is flexed forwards and rests on, or close to, the anterior cortex with insufficient cement fixation, as shown in Figure 11.5. This problem can be prevented by careful positioning during reaming and cementing, and also by the use of an intramedullary cement restrictor and injector to ensure good pressurization of the cement at the time of fixation.

In another personal series of 49 patients (Derby) followed for up to 5 years after Souter–Strathclyde elbow arthroplasty, it was noted that the radiographs of five patients demonstrated 'cement radiolucent lines' of more than 3 mm around the ulnar component, suggesting radiological evidence of loosening, although no patient had clinical evidence of loosening at the time of review.

Experience of other designs of elbow arthroplasty have shown that problems of cement fixation also occur to a varying extent in other implants, such as the Wadsworth Mark 1, Lowe and Liverpool arthroplasties, but it may be that there are some situations in which the longer stems of the Wadsworth Mark 2 and the capitellocondylar (Ewald) arthroplasties reduce the risk of poor cement fixation even though they do not have such good cortical protection against rotational stresses as the 'stirrup' design of the Souter–Strathclyde humeral component.

Loosening remains one of the main limiting factors with regard to the longevity of elbow arthroplasties and it is therefore important that patients have a realistic perception of the early limitations of their artificial joint; abuse and overuse can lead to early problems, such as in one patient who indulged in repetitive use of a 3 kg lump hammer, with detrimental effects to his elbow replacement which subsequently became loose. Therefore, clear and unequivocal joint protection rules must be given to the patient, who will naturally be tempted to

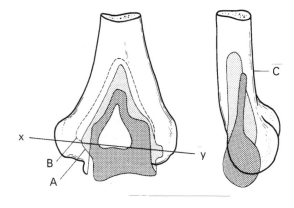

Figure 11.5 Alignment of the humeral component: position A, incomplete seating – high risk of loosening; position B, correct position; position C, incorrect – component rotated so that there is a cement deficiency anteriorly at the proximal tip of the stem. This can be difficult to identify at the time of surgery.

overuse a pain-free joint. A joint protection regimen should be provided, either verbally or in the form of a printed hand-out, or preferably both.

Implant failure

Stress fractures of the metal components or fragmentation of the ultrahigh molecular weight polyethylene (UHMWPE) is rare in our experience and is mainly confined to the constrained implants such as the elbow hinges. Some of these arthroplasties developed problems with the linkage mechanism of the hinge, resulting in loosening and sometimes complete detachment of the gudgeon pin so that the components became 'unhinged'. Later prostheses which contained different types of low-friction bearing developed problems with wear in these bearings in the early stages, although the latest designs with metal on UHMWPE have not suffered from these problems.

The Silastic flexible hinge arthroplasty also failed and is no longer used as it was found to be unable to take the stresses involved across the elbow joint.

The present trend towards less constrained implants has resulted in a much lower incidence of implant failure and the main problem is now in relation to the fixation and possible wear of the polyethylene component. There are insufficient results available at this stage to be able to do more than hypothesize, but there is certainly much debate, as there is in relation to lower limb arthroplasties, as to whether or not the polyethylene component should be cemented directly into bone or whether it should be supported in a metal 'tray'. Certainly, what has not been resolved is the problem of what happens to a polyethylene component over the years as it gradually wears, perhaps developing polyethylene granulomas (as in the hip), and in addition whether the phenomenon of 'creep' will affect wear and late loosening. It is also unclear whether or not a metal tray will improve the situation or whether the tray itself would be vulnerable to late stress fractures, as has been described in the tibial components of total knee replacements (Moran et al, 1991).

What is clear, however, is that any failure of technique, such as leaving cement fragments interposed between the implant components, or malalignment or instability of the components, is likely to lead to increased wear of the polyethylene component and subsequent loosening.

Infection

The elbow is a subcutaneous joint and is therefore vulnerable to infection, as shown in Figure 11.6. Following elbow arthroplasty, patients are at particular risk of developing deep infection of the arthroplasty if there is a failure of primary wound healing in the early postoperative stages, or the development of a pressure sore, an ulcer or olecranon bursitis at a later stage. The skin overlying the olecranon is normally very sensitive and can be pinched strongly without any severe discomfort. After an operation in this region there is inevitably partial denervation of the cutaneous nerves locally, which will reduce the skin sensibility further and render the patient vulnerable to pressure ulceration over the tip of the elbow. It is our practice, therefore, to provide all patients with a sheepskin pad which they can apply to the elbow during the first 2 months postoperatively in order to try and minimize the risk of these other problems (Figure 11.7). These risks are further increased after revision surgery when old surgical scars may well have already impaired both the nerve and blood supply to the skin in this region.

Most patients undergoing this type of surgery will be suffering from rheumatoid arthritis and, either as a result of the disease itself or as a secondary effect of the medication, will be more susceptible to infection than the average patient. Every effort needs to be made to reduce the risk of infection by careful preoperative assessment to ensure there are no septic foci present, by meticulous preoperative preparation of the skin of the arm and by the use of 'clean-air' theatres. Other measures, such as the use of prophylactic antibiotics at the time of surgery and antibiotic-loaded cement, also have a place but are probably of secondary importance.

Correct and meticulous attention to *surgical technique* will help to reduce the risks of infection at the time of surgery. It is perhaps worth emphasizing some aspects of technique which will already be well known but which are of relevance in this context, as attention to detail at this stage will reduce the likelihood of complications later.

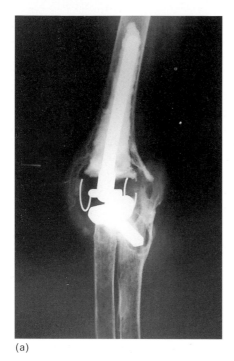

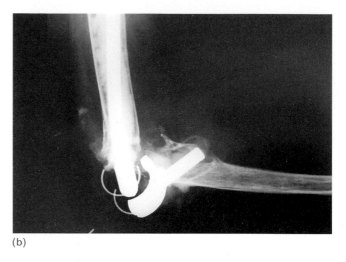

(b)

Figure 11.6 (a) AP and (b) lateral radiographs of an infected elbow arthroplasty. The patient had been treated on long-term antibiotics. The bone has resorbed and the components have loosened, thus constituting a difficult problem for revision surgery. If surgery is offered, a two-stage procedure is recommended.

(a)

Straight incisions are less likely to produce ischaemic skin flap necrosis than curved incisions; a long straight incision should avoid undue skin tension during the operation and will provide satisfactory access. The skin should not be undermined superficially; dissection should take place deep to the deep fascia in order to preserve the cutaneous blood supply. It is also important to close the deep fascia as a separate layer at the end of the operation; allowing the deep fascia to retract further diminishes the blood supply to the skin edges, often already reduced by the effect of previous surgery and rheumatoid vasculitis.

Any evidence of skin necrosis requires *emergency* excision of the necrotic skin and primary closure of the defect. In some instances local skin flap cover may be required and in view of the difficulty of achieving such cover in this region it may be necessary to seek advice and assistance from a plastic surgeon.

Patient selection

The majority of patients requiring elbow arthroplasty at the present time are those with rheumatoid arthritis. It is well recognized that this condition is associated with a reduction in the normal immune response to infection and this can be further impaired by some of the

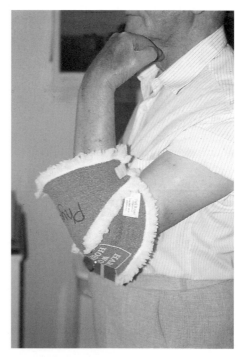

Figure 11.7 Protecting the elbow from injury and ulcers after operation with a sheepskin elbow 'protector' fitted with velcro straps.

treatment methods used, as already mentioned above. Particular care should therefore be taken in patients who are on steroid or immunosuppressant medication, those who have a past history of infective episodes, or are diabetics. The main risk in these patients is that of deep infection, and this risk may be heightened by skin problems and delayed wound healing.

Osteoporosis is another feature of rheumatoid arthritis and in severe cases may be contraindication to arthroplasty; bone cysts, tumours or bony defects for other reasons are also potential problems which may lead to failure.

Neuropathic joints caused by diabetes, syringomyelia or other causes, although not common, are likely to be associated with failure because the patient is more at risk of overloading the joint and ending up with excessive wear of the arthroplasty, instability or loosening.

Although there has been an increased interest in offering total elbow replacement for patients other than rheumatoid arthritics, such as those with primary osteoarthritis and with post-fracture deformity and arthritis, the failure rates with such pathologies is very much higher than with the rheumatoid patient and alternative methods of treatment (as discussed in Chapter 10) should be sought. If, however, elbow replacement is indeed the last resort, it should be used with caution and patients should be warned that they must limit their activities after such surgery.

The patient's attitude to total elbow replacement and the constraints associated with the joint protection programme are also relevant to the surgeon when assessing the patient's suitability for this procedure.

Choice of revision implant

Each patient's problem is unique and therefore requires its own unique solution. This applies particularly in the context of revision surgery. The first decision to be made relates to the technical problem of which type of implant is appropriate, if indeed revision to another implant is technically feasible and also appropriate to the patient's circumstances. The choices are:

- To do nothing but to provide supportive measures – perhaps to supply an orthosis.
- To refer the patient to a specialist centre

with more experience of revision arthroplasty.

- To revise to the same type of implant.
- To revise to a different type of implant.
- To revise to a custom-made implant.
- To revise to an excisional arthroplasty.

There are a variety of elbow implants available at the present time and these can be classified into the following groups.

Minimally constrained surface replacements (e.g. Liverpool, Lowe–Miller and ICLH arthroplasties)

These arthroplasties depend on the presence of good bone stock and they require minimal bone excision. The ligamentous structures must also be intact in order to maintain the stability of the joint.

Semiconstrained arthroplasties with intramedullary fixation (e.g. Souter–Strathclyde, capitellocondylar (Ewald), Wadsworth Mark II and Kudo arthroplasties)

Because of more secure fixation these arthroplasties have a wider application and can be used even in the presence of some bone erosion. It is still necessary, however, for the epicondylar ridges to be largely intact, and the stability of the joint will depend on the integrity of the soft tissues to a large extent.

Non-rigid hinge arthroplasties – also known as 'sloppy' hinges (e.g. Pritchard–Walker, Swanson hinge Coonrod-Morley)

Although these are linked hinges they allow a small amount of movement in rotational and abduction/adduction planes. This slight laxity reduces some of the stresses which are transmitted across the cement–bone interface and so should reduce the risk of loosening and bone resorption seen in the rigid hinges. These arthroplasties may well be suitable for use in some cases with more severe bone erosion and some ligamentous instability.

Rigid hinges (e.g. McKee, Dee, Shiers, Stanmore, triaxial)

Some of the earlier hinges required extensive resection of bone and this factor, coupled with the major problems with loosening, bone resorption and fractures, has meant that the indications for this type of arthroplasty are now very limited (Souter, 1973). In particular, the lack of options for subsequent salvage after failure has been the main problem with the rigid hinges and they should therefore only be used as a 'last resort' procedure in a very small number of cases where bone loss is a major problem (Figure 11.8).

Clinical situations requiring revision surgery

The most common clinical situations that are likely to arise are:

1 Simple loosening
2 Loosening with some bone loss but good ligaments
3 Loosening with major bone loss
4 Implant failure
5 Infection.

These will now be explored, with pointers to the management of each situation based on our own clinical experience.

Simple loosening

Generally this situation is best dealt with by using the same implant unless it is felt that the original choice was not appropriate, in which case an alternative implant must be chosen. For example, the use of a simple resurfacing implant in a bad grade IV joint would require revision to an implant with adequate intramedullary fixation of some type (Souter, Ewald, Wadsworth). What is essential in any case of loosening is to establish the *cause* of the loosening and ensure that any further procedures will avoid the same problem arising again (Figure 11.9).

Loosing with some bone loss but with good ligaments

The management of this situation is similar to the previous group, but some of these patients may require longer-stemmed components, which are often available as 'revision' units (Figure 11.10).

Loosening with major bone loss

Management of this situation becomes more difficult. The bone loss may be either on the humeral or the ulnar side and will usually require some form of custom-made implant to fill the bony defect and allow for adequate intramedullary fixation. Few companies offer this type of facility and, when available, it is very costly. However, in appropriate cases it is more cost effective than running the risk of further complications and a protracted hospital stay for the patient if an unsatisfactory implant is used.

Implant failure

It is rare for this to occur without bone loss. The old elbow hinges frequently failed because of loosening rather than fracture of the implant. The biomechanical stresses across an upper limb prosthesis are not nearly as large as they are in the lower limb and therefore stress fractures of the stems of the implants are much less common. More common is some form of mechanical failure, such as loosening, wear or detachment of the hinge mechanism or gudgeon pin, but as this type of rigid linked implant is rarely used nowadays the problem is rarely encountered. The solution to this type of problem will usually involve revision of the implant to a 'sloppy hinge' as long as there is sufficient bone to allow secure fixation.

Wear of the polyethylene component of the arthroplasty is likely to become a more common problem in the future. Accelerated wear will occur if there is a mechanical problem, such as malalignment of the components so that they are not articulating in a congruent manner. Cement interposition will also cause very rapid wear of the polyethylene. It is therefore important to identify whether or not there is such a predisposing cause which needs to be remedied before replacing the worm component(s).

If there is major bone loss associated with implant failure it is likely that special revision or custom-made components will be required.

Infection

Infection is not necessarily associated with major bone erosion or resorption and the same principles apply as for infection of any cemen-

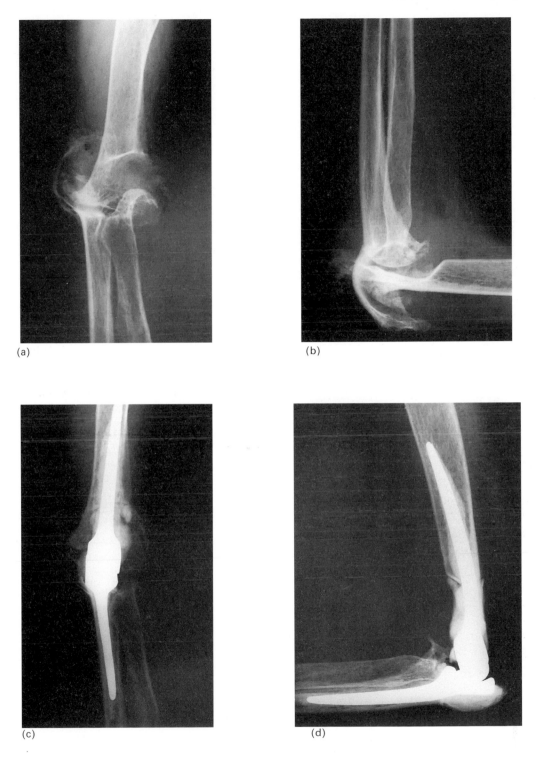

(a)

(b)

(c)

(d)

Figure 11.8 Constrained hinge arthroplasty. Preoperative radiographs: (a) AP and (b) lateral views showing gross bony erosion resulting in an unstable elbow – similar to an excisional arthroplasty. Postoperative radiographs: (c) AP and (d) lateral views after insertion of a triaxial hinged elbow arthroplasty.

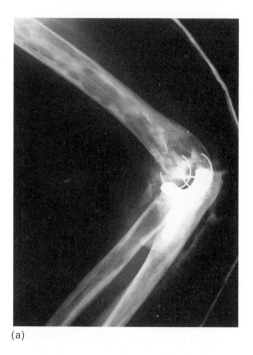

(a)

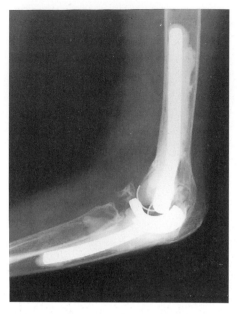

(b)

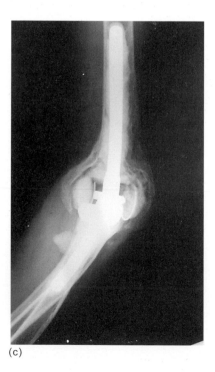

(c)

Figure 11.9 Conversion to long-stemmed 'revision' implants for prosthetic loosening. (a) Lateral radiograph showing Wadsworth Mark 1 arthroplasty which has become painful owing to loosening of the humeral component. Post-operative radiographs: (b) AP and (c) lateral views after revision with long-stemmed components.

ted joint replacement. It should be stressed, however, that the elbow is not a 'forgiving' joint in terms of its ability to combat infection and therefore a cautious approach is usually required; this may well involve a two-stage procedure with removal of the components and cement initially, followed by reinsertion of a further arthroplasty, if indicated, 3–6 months later.

However, if ligamentous instability is present in any of the situations outlined above then there are only four possible courses of action:

1 Abandon all attempts to treat the case and refer the patient to a centre with greater experience.
2 Abandon revision and leave an excisional arthroplasty.
3 Revise to an unconstrained arthroplasty with full ligament reconstruction.
4 Revise to a linked 'sloppy hinge' such as a Pritchard–Walker.

Technical aspects of revision surgery

The detailed decision-making which take place at the time of revision surgery will not be explored, focusing on the practical aspects of how revision surgery should be undertaken. This will cover:

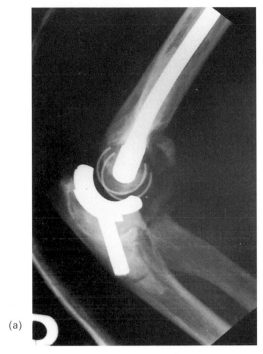 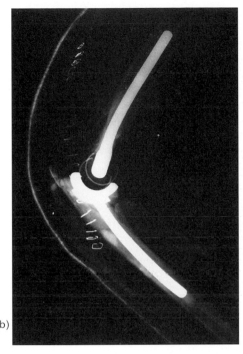

(a) (b)

Figure 11.10 Loosening of the ulnar component. (a) Lateral radiograph of short-stemmed ulnar component showing fracture of the cement close to the tip of the stem with loosening. (b) Postoperative radiograph: lateral view showing revision of the ulnar component with a long-stemmed implant.

- surgical instruments and implants
- surgical approaches
- preservation of soft tissues
- preparation of bone
- positioning of components
- cementing techniques
- salvage techniques.

Surgical instruments and implants

The need for the correct instrumentation and availability of an adequate set of implants cannot be overemphasized. It is necessary to have high-speed burrs with adequate cooling, a fibreoptic light guide, narrow offset goose-neck gouges and standard high-performance suction and irrigation facilities. A full range of elbow implants must be available, including revision components and sometimes also special custom-made components. Although the author's preference is for the Souter–Strathclyde implants, probably the correct choice will be the implant with which the surgeon has had the greatest experience.

Surgical approaches

There are three basic surgical approaches that are used for elbow arthroplasty; surgeons involved in revision surgery need to be familiar with all of these techniques as the original operation may have been carried out in another centre and it is sometimes necessary to carry out the revision using the same approach as the original operation. The various approaches are dealt with in more detail elsewhere so we will only briefly mention some of the relevant features of each approach, without describing the approach itself in detail.

Posterior approach

The Campbell posterolateral approach, in which a distally based 'tongue' of triceps is fashioned, gives good exposure of the elbow joint and probably has the lowest incidence of complications. The potential problems are due to the wound being close to the tip of the olecranon and therefore there is the risk of skin breakdown, sinus formation and possible infection. In practice this is not a major problem but may be a particular risk in patients on steroids or with other disorders leading to delayed wound healing. The transolecranon variation of the posterior approach (utilizing an osteotomy of the olecranon) has now largely been abandoned for use in elbow arthroplasty, although it may be that a modified form of the technique where a small extra-articular 'slither' of bone is taken at the triceps insertion may still be appropriate in some cases (Bryan and Morrey, 1982; Figgie et al, 1989). Problems in achieving sound bony union of the osteotomy in rheumatoid patients in the past has meant that there was a high incidence of failure of the fixation of the osteotomy in the short term and non-union in the longer term, eventually leading to loosening of the ulnar component.

Lateral approach

The extended Kocher approach has been associated with a high incidence of ulnar nerve compression complications in the past. In an early series using this approach for the capitellocondylar arthroplasty, Ewald et al (1980) reported ulnar nerve compression signs and symptoms in 11 of 64 patients, five of whom suffered permanent residual impairment of nerve conduction. Certainly, this approach does not allow good visualization of the nerve and thus the nerve is more vulnerable to traction, compression or other injury during the operation.

Medial approach

Bryan and Morrey have described a posteromedial approach in which the ulnar nerve is identified and then the triceps muscle is raised as a continuous flap from medial to lateral and from proximal to distal, raising the extensor carpi ulnaris and anconeus muscles from the ulna in continuity. This has been reported as giving good exposure as well as good wound healing and seems to protect the ulnar nerve adequately (Morrey and Bryan 1982, 1987).

Preservation of soft tissues

As has already been mentioned, the *ulnar nerve* must be protected as this is the structure at most risk during revision surgery. It is essential to identify the nerve proximally as it lies under the triceps muscle some 6–10 cm proximal to the cubital tunnel. Freeing the nerve while

preserving its 'mesentery' takes time in the primary case but even more so in the revision case; nevertheless it is vital for adequate exposure. Transposition of the nerve at the time of joint replacement has been unrewarding and in our last 150 elbow replacement operations we have not found it necessary. It is interesting to note that effective decompression of the nerve is all that is required as long as its vascularity is preserved.

It is important to preserve the anterior portion of the *medial ligament* and the annular ligament in order to maintain the stability of the joint, unless a constrained prosthesis is being used. In the unusual event of the medial ligament being deficient it will need to be reconstructed, either using a free tendon graft or with local transfer of part of the tendinous portion of the flexor muscle origin attached to the medial epicondyle. This type of reconstruction is more commonly required during secondary surgery and has already been discussed in detail above.

Preparation of bone

In order to achieve sound fixation it is important to insert the arthroplasty into secure bone. For most of the currently used prostheses, this means preservation of the epicondylar ridges. Fracture of the medial epicondyle is the most commonly encountered problem in this respect and will jeopardize the fixation of the humeral component. During revision surgery this is a particular hazard which should be avoided by careful preparation of the bone using a powered sagittal saw and burrs rather than osteotomes or gouges.

The olecranon is severely eroded in some cases and is just a thin 'eggshell' of cortical bone that can easily be fractured if it is excavated with burrs or if too much traction is applied to it. In these cases it will be necessary to use a stemmed ulnar component, probably with a metal 'tray' to support it. This is quite a common problem in revision surgery and it is important to have access to a full range of prostheses so that a suitable component may be used.

Positioning of components

Failure to achieve correct alignment of the components can result in impaired function or, at worst, may result in failure of the arthroplasty due to instability, loosening or a combination of the two. Revision surgery in this situation may be relatively easy unless the previous arthroplasty has been positioned too far medially, which is a common error and results in the medial epicondyle being very thin and fragile.

Cementing techniques

The majority of elbow arthroplasties are cemented into the bone and there is not yet sufficient evidence to suggest that uncemented techniques have any definite advantage. Where the design of the humeral component allows sufficient surface area to permit good fixation in bone there is usually no difficulty in achieving a stable cement–bone interface, although sometimes a cement restrictor will give better impaction of the cement. The ulnar component poses more problems, in that it is difficult to keep the cement under pressure during insertion. If the bone interface is deficient, loosening will almost inevitably occur (Figure 11.10).

Salvage techniques

When embarking on revision surgery it is essential to have a clear 'escape route' so that if during the operation it becomes clear that a further arthroplasty cannot be carried out, some other option is available that will nevertheless give the patient some useful function. It is also important to have discussed these possible options with the patient beforehand so that they have a realistic expectation of the results of surgery and are fully informed of the possible outcome.

If joint replacement is not possible there are only four other options, and in our view only the first of these is a practical option.

Excision arthroplasty

This procedure can result in a pain-free joint with a good and sometimes excellent range of motion. Unfortunately, after such a procedure the elbow is weak and is not suitable for lifting or weight-bearing without some form of external support. It is necessary to fashion the bone ends so that the lower end of the humerus forms a 'wishbone' structure into which the ulna can stabilize and articulate. The arm needs to be immobilized for approximately 6 weeks in order to allow the soft tissues to form a strong fibrous pseudarthrosis. Patients can usually achieve a very satisfactory range of movement and use the arm to carry out many of the tasks of normal hygiene and daily living but may require a hinged elbow orthosis for more powerful functions.

Arthrodesis

Surgical fusion of the elbow is effective in relieving elbow pain but otherwise has little to commend it. In the rheumatoid patient it is seldom, if ever, indicated as there is too great a loss of function, particularly as the shoulder and other upper limb joints are frequently also impaired and are unable to compensate for the loss of motion at the elbow.

Elbow allografting

This technique has been reported in a small number of cases but with limited success (Urbaniak, 1986). Although the procedure is technically feasible and the graft has become incorporated in several cases, there have also been cases of non-union, fractures and, perhaps more disturbing, marked bone resorption in later stages due to 'Charcot-like' changes in the joint. This procedure can therefore only be regarded as experimental at the present time.

Amputation

Even a painful unstable elbow if adequately splinted can provide a degree of function. Amputation would obviously only be considered as a last resort in very dire circumstances – perhaps in a patient with an infection which cannot be controlled. It has never been necessary in Wrightington or Derby.

Conclusions

Revision surgery of the elbow is a technique which is still very much in its infancy but it is to be hoped that, if many of the lessons already learned from lower limb arthroplasties can be applied to the upper limb, some of the worst mistakes may be avoided. Revision surgery

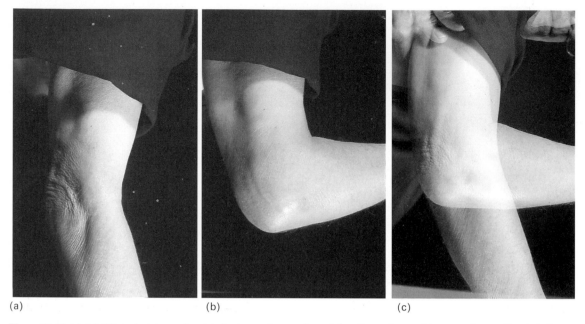

(a)   (b)   (c)

Figure 11.11 (a)–(c) Clinical pictures showing flexion and extension of the elbow after revision to a Souter–Strathclyde arthroplasty. There is slight restriction of full movement but a useful functional range.

requires a degree of experience based on previous successful treatment of a good variety of primary cases and the availability of suitable back-up resources in terms of skilled rehabilitation therapists. In view of the relatively small numbers of elbow prostheses being implanted, this experience is not widely available. Therefore the second of the surgical options identified earlier – 'abandon all attempts to treat the case and refer' – may sometimes be the wisest action to take. Certainly, the end result in any patient's elbow replacement is always related to the quality not the quantity of the operations and it is our responsibility as surgeons to develop these techniques into an increasingly precise art form which will provide our patients with a predictable and reliable result, giving both good pain relief and good function without undue risk to the patient, as shown in Figure 11.11.

References

Bryan RS and Morrey BF (1982) Extensive posterior exposure of the elbow: a triceps-sparing approach. *Clinical Orthopaedics* **166** 188–192.

Ewald FC, Scheinberg RD, Poss R, Thomas WH, Scott RD and Sledge CB (1980) Capitellocondylar total elbow arthroplasty: two to five-year follow-up in rheumatoid arthritis. *Journal of Bone and Joint Surgery* **62A** 1259–1263.

Figgie MP, Inglis AE, Mow CS and Figgie HE III (1989) Total elbow arthroplasty for complete ankylosis of the elbow. *Journal of Bone and Joint Surgery* **71A** 513–520.

Moran CG, Pinder IM, Lees PA et al (1991) Survivorship analysis of the uncemented porous-coated anatomic knee replacement. *Journal of Bone and joint Surgery* **73A** 848–857.

Morrey BF and Bryan RS (1982) Complications of total elbow arthroplasty. *Clinical Orthopaedics* **170** 204–212.

Morrey BF and Bryan RS (1987) Revision total elbow arthroplasty. *Journal of Bone and Joint Surgery* **69A** 523–532.

Morrey BF, An KN and Chao EYS (1985) Functional evaluation of the elbow. In *The Elbow and its Disorders* (BF Morrey, ed.), pp. 73–91. Philadelphia: Saunders.

Pinder I (1991) Reference on the failure of tibial plates.

Souter WA (1973) Arthroplasty of the elbow – with particular reference to metallic hinge arthroplasty in rheumatoid patients. *Orthopedic Clinics of North America* **4** 395–413.

Urbaniak JR (1986) Cadaveric elbow allografts: an eight year experience. *Journal of Bone and Joint Surgery (Br)* **68B** 676.

12

Rehabilitation after total elbow replacement

Dorcas Damrel

Severe rheumatoid disease of the elbow joint has both direct and indirect effects on the function of the upper limb. The direct effects are pain, instability, reduced range of motion and swelling. The indirect effects are related to a greater or lesser extent to the direct effects.

Pain will inhibit the use of the whole limb. Combined with instability it will reduce both the control and amount of weight which can be carried in the hand.

Loss of range of motion in extension is of less importance than loss of flexion. Loss of flexion will make all tasks where the hand has to be brought to the face more difficult, and combined with instability can make, for example, the control of a knife and fork when eating a difficult or painful manoeuvre. This can have major physical and psychological effects as it robs patients of their independence – to the rheumatoid patient a very valuable commodity.

Severe reduction in the range of pronation and supination will also reduce the functional use of the hand for a large number of tasks. Elbow replacement can only have a partial effect on the range of pronation and supination if multiple joint disease has affected the inferior radioulnar joint, but the majority of patients will have some improvement in this range.

Preoperative patient management

Before surgery the patient should be fully assessed by the team physiotherapist, with a detailed assessment of the elbow to be operated on, including range of movement, muscle power, pain and function. Assessment of the shoulder and hand is also necessary as the function of the elbow joint will be affected by the condition of the other joints of the limb.

The operative procedure and the postoperative regimen should be explained to the patient, with the reasons for the positioning of any wound drains. The patient should also be referred to the occupational therapy department for functional support and advice, including the provision of any aids to daily living that may be necessary in either the short or long term.

If a continuous passive motion (CPM) machine is to be used in the postoperative period it should be fitted to the patient before surgery. The use of a CPM machine will be discussed in a later section of this chapter.

Postoperative patient management

Treatment aims

General aims for the patient
1 To prevent immediate postoperative respiratory and circulatory complications.
2 To help with the control of postoperative pain.
Specific aims for the elbow
3 To maintain, and where possible to increase,

the preoperative range of movement, both flexion–extension and pronation–supination.
4 To restore functional use of the arm.

Methods

Prevention of immediate postoperative respiratory and circulatory complications

Routine breathing exercises are practised postoperatively, with the use of standard techniques to remove secretions from the lungs as necessary. Active hand and shoulder exercises for the operated limb will also be practised, with attention to the maintenance of circulation, mobility and strength in the limb. These can be impaired if the wound dressing is too tight, and the bandages should be adjusted as necessary.

The patient is encouraged to be ambulant as soon as practically possible after surgery. Antiembolism stockings may be worn to increase venous return if the patient's general mobility is compromised for any reason.

Control of postoperative pain

The patient will receive standard systemic analgesia as required. The physiotherapist can supplement this by various methods, for example:

- direct heat or cold therapy
- transcutaneous nerve stimulation
- electrotherapy.

Maintenance and improvement of range of movement

Active and active assisted exercises of the elbow joint can commence between 48 hours and 3 days postoperatively. The wound dressings should be sufficiently reduced to allow free movement at the elbow. Treatment using a CPM machine can now be started. Flexion–extension, pronation–supination are practised several times a day for short (10-minute) periods. A friction-free surface such as a re-education board or smooth table can be used to help the flexion and extension movements. External force which is not under the patient's control should not be applied to the elbow for up to 3 weeks after operation as this may compromise soft tissue repair. Gentle movements that are autoassisted by the patient can

be allowed as these exercises are under the patient's control.

Oedema around the elbow can restrict the range of movement and slow down the recuperative process. We have used the following methods (in order of frequency) to control and reduce oedema, either alone or in conjunction.

1 Simple elevation of the limb.
2 Ice packs or cold packs.
3 Graduated Tubigrip extending from the metacarpophalangeal joints to the axilla.
4 The Flowtron apparatus.

Exercise of the joint may have to be interrupted if wound healing is not satisfactory. This can be due to increased fluid leakage, haematoma, delayed skin healing or infection. The wound should be inspected regularly, and if any of these conditions are present physiotherapy treatment should be modified according to the patient's progress.

When the joint range, muscle power and pain control of the elbow are adequate, the patient can start using the arm in unstressed activities, for instance self-care, eating, turning book or magazine pages. This can be from around 5–10 days postoperatively, depending on the condition of both the elbow and the other joints of the limb.

The occupational therapist will play an increasingly important part in the rehabilitation of the patient from this stage as free exercise gives way to functional activities.

Restoration of functional use of the arm

Close co-operation between the physiotherapist and occupational therapist is instrumental in achieving the maximum potential from the patient following surgery. Exercises and activities directed towards the patient's goals are continued and the activity level increased as the patient improves in function.

Resisted exercises to increase muscle power and endurance can be gradually introduced from 4 weeks after surgery.

An approximate guide to the resumption of various activities is given on below.

Household tasks:	light dusting 4 weeks
	vacuuming 6 weeks
Gardening:	light weeding 6 weeks
	digging – not recommen-

	ded until at least 3 months but in general should be avoided, after elbow replacement
Driving	8 weeks - but must be confirmed by the surgeon
Lifting and carrying:	hardback book 3 weeks full 2-pint (1-litre) saucepan 6 weeks heavy shopping – not recommended until at least 3 months but in general should be avoided after elbow replacement.

A successful outcome from total elbow replacement will include both a reduction of pain and an improvement in the functional use of the arm. It is important that the patient is aware that the operation does not restore normality to the joint and that undue stresses and strains may reduce the lifetime of the joint and contribute to loosening or damage of the components. Patients with severe multijoint disease affecting other joints of the upper limb will be less likely to abuse the elbow as overuse of this joint will cause pain in the other affected joints.

Patients with normal or minimally affected hand, wrist and shoulder joints need careful education about the limitations of elbow joint replacements and should be encouraged to take partial responsibility for a successful long-term result from surgery.

Use of a constant passive motion machine after total elbow replacement

The use of a constant passive motion (CPM) machine is usually started between 2 and 5 days postoperatively after X-ray and once the wound has been checked.

The machine will have been fitted to the patient preoperatively, with any extra padding attached to the handgrip as required. Patients with severe rheumatoid disease causing hand and/or wrist deformities can have difficulties with the fitting of the CPM machine, but the judicious use of extra padding will overcome this.

Postoperatively, the range of motion of the CPM machine is set to the patient's pain-free range of flexion and extension. Care should be taken with the flexion range so that the triceps aponeurosis repair is not compromised. The aim of the treatment is to obtain the range of motion of the elbow that was achieved on the operating table, but this is often not regained until the postoperative swelling has subsided.

The CPM machine is initially applied for short periods several times a day, for example 30–45 minutes three times a day, depending on the patient's tolerance and pain level. The time spent on the machine can be gradually increased over the ensuing days. The range of motion is increased by setting the machine to coincide with the patient's range of motion, as this increases. *The CPM machine should not be used to manipulate the elbow with either further flexion or further extension than the patient can achieve unaided.*

If use of CPM causes a definite increase in the patient's pain level it should be removed and the pain allowed to settle. The CPM treatment can then be recommenced, but if the pain returns it may mean that CPM should be discarded completely for that particular patient.

Use of CPM may have to be temporarily curtailed if there is an unacceptable amount of oedema in the arm and hand as a result of the arm being dependent. The range of CPM movement should not be set at a range which causes visible tension on the suture line as this may compromise wound healing.

In the author's experience the use of a CPM is most beneficial in the early stages after surgery, that is the first 10–14 days. After this CPM may be useful in the morning exercise session to maintain the range of movement achieved the previous day. The afternoon can be used to practise active exercises to increase the range of movement. Once patients can maintain their own range of movement the use of CPM should be discontinued.

Index